The
AD/HD Book

THE
AD/HD BOOK

· ·

Answers to Parents' Most Pressing Questions

· ·

Beth Ann Hill

with

James A. Van Haren, M.D., FRCPC

AVERY
a member of
Penguin Group (USA) Inc.
New York

AVERY

Published by the Penguin Group
Penguin Group (USA) Inc., 375 Hudson Street, New York, New York 10014, USA ·
Penguin Group (Canada), 90 Eglinton Avenue East, Suite 700, Toronto, Ontario M4P 2Y3, Canada
(a division of Pearson Penguin Canada Inc.) · Penguin Books Ltd, 80 Strand, London
WC2R 0RL, England · Penguin Ireland, 25 St Stephen's Green, Dublin 2, Ireland (a division of
Penguin Books Ltd) · Penguin Group (Australia), 250 Camberwell Road, Camberwell, Victoria 3124,
Australia (a division of Pearson Australia Group Pty Ltd) · Penguin Books India Pvt Ltd,
11 Community Centre, Panchsheel Park, New Delhi–110 017, India · Penguin Group (NZ),
Cnr Airborne and Rosedale Roads, Albany, Auckland 1310, New Zealand (a division of Pearson
New Zealand Ltd) · Penguin Books (South Africa) (Pty) Ltd, 24 Sturdee Avenue,
Rosebank, Johannesburg 2196, South Africa

Penguin Books Ltd, Registered Offices: 80 Strand, London WC2R 0RL, England

Library of Congress Cataloging-in-Publication Data

Hill, Beth Ann.
The AD/HD book : answers to parents' most pressing questions /
Beth Ann Hill with James Van Haren.
p.   cm.
Includes bibliographical references and index.
ISBN 1-58333-233-2
1. Attention-deficit hyperactivity disorder—Popular works.   2. Attention-deficit hyperactivity
disorder—Miscellanea.   I. Title: Attention-deficit hyperactivity disorder book.
II. Van Haren, James.   III. Title.
RJ506.H9H547   2005   2005045260
618.92'8589—dc22

Printed in the United States of America
1   3   5   7   9   10   8   6   4   2

Book design by Amanda Dewey

To my three lovely children

Acknowledgments

I would like to thank the following individuals and organizations for their help with obtaining research and for the inspiration needed to write the book:

- My editors, Kristen Jennings and Rebecca Behan, for their tremendous help and insight
- Dr. James Van Haren for spending so much of his time helping to write and edit the book (and for the wonderful foreword)
- My mother, Shirley Jo Praed, for teaching me through example
- The following individuals for helping edit the book and for their valuable suggestions—Dr. Steven Hinshaw, Dr. Oren Mason, Dr. Peter Safer, and Dr. Julie T. Steck
- The following teachers and school personnel for their love and support of our children—Scott Korpak, Diane Wickliff, Jeanne Schierloh, Kathy Ecclesine, Jim Barber, Stacey Mullen, Trudy Vyverman, Sue Laurie, Audrey Hess, Kim Fowler, Nancy Lass, Nancy Keck, Eileen Cook, Lynn Greer, Khrista Kohlhaas, Jean Lewis, Maureen Ward, Pat Wooley, Amy Forslund Amos, Joe Payne, Alisha Sage, Suzy Douma, Jenny Craffey, Cathy Maki, Maureen Milanowski,

Bruce Vorce, Barb Bigari, Sandy Baxter, Irene Pratt, Rita Dykhouse, Sarah Boer, Melissa Smith, Carol Jewell, Marcia Olsen, Jill Turner, Cindy Fedewa, and Laura Beach

- The staff members at DeVos Children's Hospital's AD/HD Intervention Program for their insight on sensory issues
- The following individuals for their tremendous help on the pharmaceutical issues of medication use—Denise Brasheer, Novartis Pharmaceuticals Corporation; Stuart Arbuckle and Heleen DeCory, Celltech; Kuleni Gebisa, Fleishman Hillard, McNeil Consumer Drugs & Specialty Pharmaceuticals; and Rob Smith and Jennifer Gremmels, Eli Lilly and Company.

Contents

· ·

CHAPTER 1. UNDERSTANDING AD/HD   1

What is attention-deficit/hyperactivity disorder (AD/HD)? • What is a "disorder"? Is AD/HD a disease? • I've seen attention-deficit/hyperactivity disorder listed as ADD, ADHD, and AD/HD. Which abbreviation is correct? • Does AD/HD really exist? • Why is AD/HD so controversial? • What areas of the brain are affected by AD/HD? • What areas of behavior and learning do these affected areas of the brain control? • Why can't scientists use neuroimaging to determine whether an individual has AD/HD? • What is the connection between dopamine and AD/HD? • What causes AD/HD? • Does genetics play a major role in the development of AD/HD? • Can bad parenting cause AD/HD? • Can other disorders be confused with AD/HD? • Can other disorders go along with AD/HD? What are these disorders? • Is AD/HD related to Asperger's disorder or autism? • Is AD/HD caused by a food or chemical allergy? • How common is AD/HD in children? • Can a child grow out of AD/HD? • Can AD/HD be cured? • Has the number of people with AD/HD gone up in the past few years? • How does AD/HD affect our society? How does it affect AD/HD children? • Why is it so important to treat AD/HD?

CHAPTER 5. ALTERNATIVE PRACTICES 60

What about special diets to treat AD/HD? • What about vitamins and minerals to treat AD/HD? • What about the use of medicinal herbs to treat AD/HD? • What about other complementary and alternative practices?

CHAPTER 6. COPING WITH THE DIAGNOSIS 64

Should I tell my child that he or she has AD/HD? • How can I help my child cope with AD/HD? • Should I spend extra time with my AD/HD child? • Are there any children's books about AD/HD that you would recommend for my child? • My teenager has just been diagnosed with AD/HD. How can I help him cope? • Are there any books that you would recommend for my AD/HD teen? • My child's grandparents don't understand. They just think he is misbehaving. How do I help them understand AD/HD? • Should I tell other people that my child has AD/HD? • Taking my AD/HD child to the grocery is a nightmare. She touches and asks for everything. How can I make this easier? • I'm losing my mind with my AD/HD child or teenager. How do I personally cope with this disorder? • Our child's AD/HD is creating problems in our marriage. What should we do? • What organizations are available to help with our child's AD/HD?

CHAPTER 7. EDUCATIONAL ISSUES 79

What are my child's legal rights? • What is an IEP? • Does my AD/HD child have to be placed in a special classroom? • How can I help my child's teacher understand his AD/HD? • What should I do if my child's teacher is not supportive?

CHAPTER 8. LIFESTYLE ISSUES 87

Doing homework with my child is a nightmare. How can we make this easier? • My child is constantly forgetting to bring his homework home. What should I do? • My child is too rough with his siblings, friends, and pets. What can we do? • What safety issues should we be aware of with our AD/HD child? • My child has trouble making and keeping friends. How can we help her socially? • Do AD/HD teenagers have a higher risk of developing substance problems? • Should someone with AD/HD drink alcoholic beverages? • Are there any issues with driving a car with which we should be concerned? • Should our AD/HD teen be allowed to babysit?

Foreword

AD/HD has been in the medical literature since the late nineteenth century. The children were described as hyperactive, having behavior problems, and being unable to concentrate. At the time, the disorder was believed to be caused by a deficit in moral control. After similar behavior was observed in children who survived encephalitis (following the 1918 influenza pandemic), it was believed that an "organic" cause was responsible for these children's difficulties. The term "minimal brain damage" was coined. As there were concerns about the connotation of brain damage, this was later modified to "minimal brain dysfunction" (MBD). Later, researchers noticed inattention and poor impulse control were more central than hyperactivity, and the term *attention-deficit disorder*—with or without hyperactivity—was used. Today, the terminology is *attention-deficit/hyperactivity disorder,* with three subtypes: primarily inattentive (AD/HD-I), primarily hyperactive/impulsive (AD/HD-HI), and combined subtype (AD/HD-C).

All children show symptoms of AD/HD at times. And with the changes in terminology, many parents are confused and bewildered over the diagnosis. Most parents do not have difficulties accepting the disorder when their child is hyperactive (although some will ask, "Isn't this just normal *childhood* behavior?"). Many struggle to understand how their son or daughter could have this diagnosis when they are able to watch cartoons for hours. Other parents are guilt-ridden, feeling they are at fault with their parenting techniques, causing their child's problem. Many are uncertain as to what constitutes adequate treatment. Most are concerned about medication, believing it is "drugging" their child to control his or her behavior with medication.

With these, and the multitude of other questions parents have, Beth Ann Hill has undertaken the task of writing a comprehensive book on AD/HD. Besides sharing the journey her family has experienced with AD/HD, she has also thoroughly researched the topic and condensed the scientific literature into a very readable book for parents and teachers.

Beth has written a book that is balanced and comprehensive and honestly answers questions that parents and teachers have about this difficult disorder. Besides the extensive question-and-answer sections, she details the multimodal treatment plan for parents in Chapter 9. In Chapter 10, she gives numerous coaching lessons for parents and counselors. *The AD/HD Book* concludes with sample charts for parents and teachers.

The AD/HD Book provides answers to difficult questions and provides a solid, multimodal treatment plan for the successful management of AD/HD in children and teens.

James A. Van Haren, M.D., FRCPC
Child, Adolescent, and General Psychiatry
Grand Rapids, Michigan

Introduction

Isn't it amazing the lessons life can teach you? I remember my first experience with AD/HD. Before I was married and had three children of my own (two of them with AD/HD), I worked as a teacher. I was fresh out of college and my mind was full of all kinds of creative and unique ideas for teaching children. I believed, at the time, that I could handle anything that came my way. My oh my, the innocence of youth!

Well, my very first day of teaching was an interesting, enjoyable, frustrating and humbling experience. I was a middle-school music teacher and I taught sixth-, seventh- and eighth-graders. (You know, the squirrelly age!) The first class was a handful, anyway. We had fifty boys and girls who had signed up for choir. Most of them had never been in a choir before, and they didn't know what to expect. The girls were giggling and whispering among themselves. One young lady was applying lip gloss as she eyed the group of boys at one side. The boys were nervous. They were in the minority at the beginning, and I think more than a few of them wondered if they had made a mistake. Most of the boys sat there in silence, clearing their voices in exaggerated bass tones and glancing at the girls. A few of the boys were playing with Matchbox cars—which one of them had sneaked in.

Then there was Tom. He arrived late, threw open the door, and in a loud voice proclaimed, "Whew! I'm here!" He then proceeded to push his way past students to a rear seat. Every five minutes, there was a new disruption from Tom. He burped. He fell out of his seat, more than once. He sang loudly off-key. He jumped up, without my asking him, to help pass out music. I remember going back to my small office (actually a closet with a desk) and rubbing my brow against an oncoming headache.

I tried everything that week with Tom. I assigned seats and moved him to the front. I moved him to sit between two quiet and well-behaved students. (After a week next to him, they too started acting out.) I had him sit in the hallway. I talked with him privately. After two weeks, I met with his parents. When I began to explain his behavior, his mother told me that Tom was hyperactive (this was twenty years ago when the disorder was relatively new to most people). She then threw up her hands and said, "We just don't know what to do with him! We've tried everything!" I remember thinking at the time that Tom's parents just didn't know how to discipline their child. (I was young and a bit stupid, and perhaps a bit—no, very arrogant at the time!)

Tom and I grew together that year. I read everything I could on his disorder. I developed a star sheet for him, and when he earned a certain number of stars from me, he got an award of some sort. I also made him my assistant. He passed out music, erased the chalkboard, and helped me with all kinds of tasks. I also thought it would help the students, both musically and responsibility-wise, to see what it was like being a teacher. Once a week, for ten minutes, a student in the class would lead the group. I was surprised at how well many of them did! When Tom began his lesson, he started out by being silly (which I fully expected). I laughed, too, at his joke and then said, "Okay, Tom. You're a really funny guy, but let's get serious now. I want to see what a great job you can do." He then pulled out a worksheet that he had prepared himself and began to teach the class. I was amazed. The whole time, Tom stood very straight and talked with a calm, strong voice. Every once in a while, he would look at me and I would wink or give him a small thumbs-up.

That day was a real beginning for Tom. After his "teaching" experience, his behavior began to improve. He still had problems keeping quiet or staying in his seat, but he and I had signals to each other. When he would get too loud or disruptive, I would put my hand on his shoulder or I would say his name quietly. He would then give me a thumbs-up or a wink to let me know he understood. If things were moving too slowly for him, he would look at me with an exasperated look and shake his hands. "I think we need a little break, kids," I would say. "Everybody stand up and we are going to do a little bit of aerobics!" His face would beam and he would give me another thumbs-up.

The year went on like this. I remember one day the principal pulled me out of class briefly to ask me something. "Tom," I said. "Would you lead the class on this song?" I then stepped out of the class. The principal looked at me in disbelief. "Are you crazy? He's the worst kid in the school!" "I might be crazy," I answered. "But take a look!" We opened the door a crack, and there was Tom, conducting the class and they were singing their hearts out. I think the principal might have even forgotten what he was coming to tell me, because he walked away shaking his head.

But the real challenge for both Tom and me came in the spring. Every year, the music teacher was required to hold auditions and prepare a spring musical. When we held tryouts, Tom was there. He did a wonderful job. He was a wonderful actor, which every teacher in the school already knew. He also had a beautiful voice. When the auditions were finished, the other two teachers and I began to debate. There was no doubt that Tom was the best choice musically and dramatically for the lead. But what about his behavior? Would he even come to rehearsals? Could we depend on him?

That night, I called Tom at home. I told him that he had the lead but there were conditions. He would need to come to every rehearsal and we would have a star chart. Each day, he had to receive a star from *each* of his other teachers in order to participate in the musical. There was silence from him for a moment. "That will be awfully hard for me," he sighed. "Yes, I know," I said. "Very, very hard. But I believe in you." "I'll do it!" he practically yelled into the phone.

And true to his word, Tom behaved very well. For the next six weeks, he practically "sat on his hands," one teacher told me. He earned his stars, and every day at rehearsal, he would proudly show me his chart. The night of the performance was beautiful. The show was lovely, and Tom's face beamed the entire time. Tom's parents and grandparents and aunts and uncles and I think about everyone his parents knew in the world were sitting in the front row.

Of course, after the show, Tom began to regress slightly. He still worked hard to behave and pay attention in my class, but in other classes, he reverted to being the class clown. I talked to him about this. "I just can't help it," he said. "It's just so hard for me. By the time I think I shouldn't do something, I've already done it!"

I don't know where Tom is now or how he is doing. The year he graduated from middle school, I also moved on in my life. I left the school that summer, moved to another state, and got married. But I will never forget my last day with choir. Many of the students gave me hugs or cards. One girl brought in flowers. But Tom said nothing. As a matter of fact, he was strangely and uncharacteristically silent. When the bell rang, all the students filed out. I was starting to get things ready for the next class when I heard a noise behind me. I turned and there was Tom. "Miss Praed?" he said. (That was my maiden name.) "Yes, Tom?" I asked. He then whipped a small camera out of his pocket and quickly snapped a picture. Then with a big grin, he ran silently from the classroom.

Out of all my years teaching, I remember Tom the most. I don't know where he is, but I think about him from time to time. I hope he is happy and productive. And I hope that somehow his years as a student in my choir were helpful to him.

After my first year of teaching with Tom, I worked as a teacher for over ten years. I taught hundreds of children in Indiana, Virginia, and Michigan. During those years, I taught many, many children with AD/HD. After ten years as a teacher, I changed careers and went into public relations and crisis management. As much as I *thought* I knew about the disorder from my experiences as a teacher, I would get a "baptism by fire" when my daughters* were born. They both have AD/HD.

My older daughter, Theresa, was what they call a "blue baby." She was born with the umbilical cord around her neck. As a baby, she was very fussy and cried a great deal. She didn't sleep much and was constantly in motion.

---

*Names have been changed to protect the family's privacy.

As she grew, we constantly joked about how "high-energy" she was. My husband even played a little joke on me about this. I came back from the grocery store one day, and there she was in her walker with her hair moussed straight up. He had put on some hard rock music at top volume (we're jazz and classical fans only), and she was bouncing up and down with this wild look on her face and sky-high hair. At day care, she was constantly on the go. One day, the day-care provider brought in a photographer to take professional portraits of the children for their parents. Theresa's class photo is unique. Apparently the teachers and photographer tried for nearly an hour to get the shot. Finally, they took one. There they all are: five little toddlers dressed in their Sunday best, sitting crisscross, applesauce on the rug, and one other child—our child—sprinting out of the photo. Even then we didn't have a clue. "There she goes again," we said when we saw the picture.

When Theresa was four, we placed her in a part-time preschool run by a group of nuns. The facility had a long waiting list and was highly regarded in the city. After just a month, we were called in for a meeting with the nuns. At the meeting, they began to go on about how she didn't pay attention, wouldn't sit still during circle time, and was a disruption to the other students. As I listened, it finally began to dawn on me. "You're kicking her out, aren't you?" I asked. "Yes," the nun slowly responded. I couldn't believe it and I looked at Danny with a worried look on my face. *If the nuns couldn't handle her, then who could?* "Is there anything that we can do?" we asked. "Yes, she should be tested for AD/HD," they said. They told us if we put her on medication, they would accept her back, but only then.

So we began the long process of having her evaluated for AD/HD. We made an appointment at a well-known medical facility near our home. It had a six-week waiting period. During that time, we filled out piles of paperwork, which asked all kinds of questions. "At what week was she born? Were there any difficulties during labor? How long does she sleep each night? Was she difficult to potty-train? Does she maintain eye contact when spoken to? Does she get along with other children? Is she too rough with her play? Is she constantly on the go? Does she have any nervous tics or vocalizations?" The list went on and on. We had to get all sorts of medical information from the obstetrician who delivered her and medical records from our pediatrician. We also had to have the nuns fill out forms on her and their observations.

Finally, the day of her evaluation arrived. I took Theresa for her appointment with the pediatric psychiatrist. He greeted us and welcomed us into his office. It was a pleasant room with many plants and a large window ledge. Immediately, Theresa raced across the room and with two bounds, jumped from a large leather chair up onto the window ledge. I was mortified. "Oh Theresa," I said as I raced across the room to get her down. "You shouldn't do that." The doctor seemed unfazed as he sat down behind his desk and began to write. "Don't worry about it," he said. "You know, that window ledge is a pretty good indicator of AD/HD. Children with AD/HD who come in here can't help but jump on that ledge. Children who don't have the disorder don't jump on the ledge." He put his pen down and looked at me. "You see, children without AD/HD may *want* to jump up on the ledge, but they are able to think quickly enough that they had better not do it. By the time an AD/HD child comes to the same conclusion, they have already impulsively jumped on the ledge. I find that ledge to be a very good unofficial indicator."

After three visits with the pediatric psychiatrist, he diagnosed Theresa with AD/HD and prescribed medication. But Danny and I were reluctant. The psychiatrist told us that Theresa was the youngest child he had ever diagnosed with AD/HD. This made us very nervous. We didn't want to put her on medication—and at such a young age! We had to be bad parents to even think of such a thing! So we decided to get a second opinion. This time, we made an appointment with another well-regarded child psychologist in town. Again, we filled out a ton of paperwork for him. He then met with Theresa, once a week for eight weeks. He reviewed the paperwork, gave her intelligence tests and a battery of other ability tests, and talked with us. Finally, after two months, he told us, "Yes, the first physician was right. She is a very bright, sweet, and loving little girl, as well as being *extremely* AD/HD." I went home, went down to the basement, got on my knees, and cried.

And so, at age four, she was put on medication. We immediately began to notice a difference. She began to have tantrums less often. Instead of three or four a day, she began to have only one a day, right after her medication wore off. The nuns said they noticed a difference too. She was able to sit quietly in a group and to follow directions.

And yet we, and especially me, were distraught over giving her medication. When summer came and her time with the nuns was over, we took her off the meds. She was to start kindergarten in the fall. We thought we would wait to see how she did. We decided not to say a word to the teachers at the new school about the AD/HD diagnosis.

The first week of kindergarten went well. Theresa had a wonderful, kind teacher. Danny and I were confident that the AD/HD thing must have been some kind of big mistake.

The second week of kindergarten, Theresa and her class went on their first field trip. They took a lovely fall trip to the apple orchard. Unfortunately, neither Danny nor I could accompany the class for that trip. We both were working at the time and had important meetings. I was in my meeting when the secretary came in and told me there was an emergency call from my daughter's school. I excused myself and went quickly to the phone. "Mrs. Hill?" the principal asked. "We've lost Theresa. She has been missing for nearly an hour now." I hung up and with a wild dash, bolted from the meeting and zoomed off to the orchard. By the time I arrived there, they had found her casually strolling through the many rows of trees. She had followed a rabbit she had seen and was "having a 'venture,'" she joyfully explained.

Danny and I rationalized it. Any young child could wander off on a field trip, couldn't they? It was her first field trip and maybe she didn't know any better (even though we had told her repeatedly to stay with the group). We decided that one of us would go on all field trips with her in the future. We thought we had everything under control.

The next week, we got another call from the principal. Theresa had thrown an eraser in class. I went in and had a conference with both the principal and the teacher about Theresa's behavior. During that meeting, Theresa hid under a table. She knew she was in trouble. "Has she been tested for AD/HD?" they asked. Yes, I explained, but I still wasn't convinced. So the school evaluated her and we took her to yet *another* child psychiatrist. Both the school and the third doctor confirmed that she definitely had AD/HD.

Danny and I didn't fill the prescription for two weeks. We didn't want to do it. We argued as a couple. We read everything we could get our hands on. We still couldn't decide what was the best thing to do for her.

In November, I got another emergency call at work from Theresa's teacher. They had been working on an art project with little white beads and Theresa had put some up her nose. I again left work to go get her. When we arrived at the pediatrician's office, he took a suction device and sucked the beads from her nostrils. There were two beads in one nostril and three in the other. It was a pretty unpleasant procedure for her. All the way home in the car, she was silent. This was very unlike her; she usually talked nonstop. "Theresa, are you okay?" I asked. "Yes," she answered. And then after a long pause, she said, "You know, Mommy, that was a very bad idea."

I went home, down to the basement again. I thought about it, prayed a lot, and cried again. Finally, Danny and I decided to put her on medication.

Immediately, we noticed a difference at home. Dinnertime had been a circus before the meds. Both girls would frequently jump up from their chairs to retrieve a toy or paper they wanted to show us. Neither child really sat on a chair. When Theresa was on the meds, she actually *sat*. Before that time, she crouched, squatting on the seat as if to propel herself in flight.

Things improved at school also. Theresa had a wonderful kindergarten teacher, Mrs. Laura Beach. She set up a "stoplight" system with Theresa. Every day, Theresa would receive a green card, a yellow card, or a red card for staying on task. If Theresa received a certain number of green cards, Mrs. Beach would take her and a friend of her choice to McDonald's for lunch.

Two years later, Jenny started kindergarten with Mrs. Beach. For Jenny, kindergarten was a joy. But at the end of kindergarten, Mrs. Beach expressed concern over Jenny's academic level. Jenny was the youngest in her class and was behind in her reading ability. She also was showing signs of AD/HD. When Jenny started first grade, the pressure began to mount and Jenny began to be discouraged. She would cry nightly, saying she was sick and couldn't go to school the next day. The third week of school, I got a call from her teacher. Apparently Jenny had made an obscene gesture at another student. "That's impossible," I replied. But I told the teacher that

I would talk to Jenny when she got home. Later that day, when Jenny and I were doing homework, I asked her about it. "Did you do something with your hand?" I asked. Yes, she did and she showed me what it was. "Where did you learn that gesture?" I asked. "From the big boys at school. They do it when they're mad," she explained. "And what does it mean?" I tried to ask calmly. "It means 'I'm the boss!'" my innocent little daughter answered.

This was only the beginning. Jenny became more and more anxious. She wasn't keeping up with the other students and they were teasing her about it. The teacher called frequently, saying Jenny wasn't paying attention and would hyperfocus at times.

In November, I received a call from the principal, "Mrs. Hill? We've lost Jenny." Apparently, she had asked to go to the bathroom and hadn't returned. The principal, the librarian, the school counselor, and the janitor had looked for her, but after 45 minutes, she was still missing. As I drove to the school, I was worried. *Had she left school?* I thought. I also had a strong feeling of déjà vu. *Hadn't I been through this same situation before?* When I arrived at school, the school staff had found her. She hadn't wanted to do her reading assignment, so she had hidden in her locker. The janitor was searching for her and saw the locker move. When I walked in, she was hiding under the same table her sister had used. Even though I was very angry with her, even though I had been scared out of my wits that she was missing, I felt really sorry for her. I gathered her up in my arms and just rocked her for a few minutes in silence. "I would like to have Jenny tested for AD/HD," the principal told me. I nodded in agreement.

Jenny was diagnosed with AD/HD in December. In February, she was also diagnosed with learning disabilities in reading. In the meantime, she continued to cry and refused to go to school. Danny and I worried about her and decided that a change was due.

We did research on the area. We looked at neighborhoods, churches, and schools. We interviewed principals about their school's atmosphere and their philosophies of education. Finally, we chose a grade school in the area with an excellent reputation. We then began looking for property in that school district on which to build a house.

The following year, both girls were in the new school system. We love their current elementary school. The teachers are all highly qualified, the principal is supportive, and the secretaries are kind and understanding. Theresa and Jenny both love school now. They both still take their medications and they both need extra help and support. I tutor both girls nightly, and Jenny is in a special reading class. Theresa's teacher has a reward system where she earns marbles (which she collects) for staying on task and for transitioning quickly between activities. Both girls are in Girl Scouts. They also have participated in numerous activities—community theater, gymnastics, dance, and swimming lessons.

I am proud of my daughters. Theresa is interested in life and is an avid reader. She loves doing new things. Currently, she is interested in horses. She also is an incredible artist. Jenny is my "girly-girl" who loves dressing up and looking pretty. She also helps me a lot around the house and with her younger brother. She is very athletic and loves to dance. She has a wonderful sense of humor.

There have been many times that I have worried about them and their AD/HD. *What will they do when they are adults? How will the AD/HD affect them? Am I doing the right things now to help them? Will they grow up to be good people?* I sometimes find myself uttering the exact same words that I heard from Tom's parents more than twenty years ago: "I just don't know what to do! I've tried everything!"

I believe that it is possible for children with AD/HD, and adults too, to live happy and productive lives. The challenge is to learn how to manage the disorder and to uncover those special qualities that each of us has. People with AD/HD are often tremendously bright. They have boundless energy (something I wish I had) and are incredibly creative. What we need to do as parents is to learn how to channel those strengths in our AD/HD children, while helping them learn to manage and control the symptoms of AD/HD. I hope that this book will help you to do just that.

AD/HD is a very complicated disorder. Some speculate that it doesn't even exist. In an effort to help my girls, I have read every book on AD/HD that I could get my hands on. I've spent hundreds of hours on the Internet, talked with numerous parents in the same situation, and spent countless hours with physicians and psychiatrists. I, too, have ridden the "yes medication/no medication" merry-go-round.

In some ways, I have had an advantage. I have a master's degree in education and I had a great deal of experience with AD/HD students before my children were even born. I had the great fortune of being raised in a household with very wise and loving parents. My brother, Scott, is autistic. In a time when little was known about autism, my mother set the whole family out on a journey of learning and compassion. Single-handedly, she battled the school system in my hometown for special services for my brother. She also arranged for each one of us in the family to coach Scott daily on various tasks—a skill that I have applied in this book for AD/HD children. I am very grateful to my mom. I also have the advantage of having worked in crisis management. If having an AD/HD child isn't a crisis, I don't know what is! This book is written as a crisis manual as such. It will attempt to answer any questions that you might have, as well as giving advice on what to do and specific coaching lessons for your child.

The AD/HD Book is organized into ten chapters. The first eight are question-and-answer chapters and include Understanding AD/HD, Symptoms of AD/HD, Diagnosis and Tests, Medication, Alternative Practices, Coping with the Diagnosis, Educational Issues, and Lifestyle Issues. Next come two of the most important sections of the book: Pulling It All Together—The AD/HD Pyramid and Coaching Assignments. The final section includes charts, a driver's contract for teens, a glossary, and an extensive resource section for your information.

1.

UNDERSTANDING AD/HD

. . . .

Someone once asked me what I thought was the most important factor in helping an AD/HD child. I said, "The *second* most important factor is medication. The number-one factor in helping an AD/HD child? Parent education about AD/HD."

AD/HD is a complicated disorder—often difficult to diagnose and always difficult to understand. Being a parent is hard enough! Often we feel overextended and exhausted. Having a child with AD/HD can cause us to despair, thinking, "I don't understand this! I don't know what to do!"

I've been there. I've said and thought the same things. I hope that this beginning chapter will help you take the first step—understanding AD/HD.

What is attention-deficit/hyperactivity disorder (AD/HD)?

Attention-deficit/hyperactivity disorder is categorized as a mental or behavioral disorder. Those who have AD/HD have abnormal levels of inattention and/or hyperactivity and impulsivity.

According to the American Psychiatric Association, there are three diagnostic subtypes of AD/HD: predominantly inattentive type, or AD/HD-I (previously known as "ADD"); predominantly hyperactive-impulsive type, or AD/HD-HI; and a combined type, or AD/HD-C (previously known as "ADHD"). Those with the inattentive type of AD/HD tend to have more academic problems in school, while the hyperactive-impulsive type experience more behavior problems.

Those with AD/HD often have problems with academic achievement and social relationships. Families with an AD/HD child experience more discord and arguments. In addition, children with AD/HD are often rejected by their peers and can experience lower levels of self-esteem as a result. There is also evidence that AD/HD children experience accidental injuries more often than children without AD/HD. Unfortunately, studies have also shown that teenagers and adults with AD/HD, especially those who have not received medication and treatment, have higher levels of substance abuse, unemployment, criminal histories, and school dropout rates.

According to the Centers for Disease Control and Prevention, AD/HD is one of the most common and serious health conditions, affecting 3 percent to 7 percent of children (some experts put the percentages at 5 to 10 percent) in the United States and costing consumers $3.5 to $4 billion in the health care, education, and juvenile justice arenas.

What is a "disorder"? Is AD/HD a disease?

No, AD/HD is not a disease. A disease is a pathological condition in the body as a result of an infection or virus (for example, AIDS, diphtheria, and measles), a genetic defect (for example, cystic fibrosis), or an environmental cause, such as cancer caused by smoking, or Lyme disease, caused by the spirochete organism transmitted from ticks.

In medical terms, the word *disorder* means that there is a problem or a condition within the body that is not in the normal range of function. AD/HD is categorized as a *mental* disorder, because the problem is associated with deficits in the brain.

In years past, there was quite a bit of fear and misunderstanding about mental disorders and diseases. Today, we now know that many problems can occur in the brain. A chemical abnormality in the brain can cause depression and anxiety. Actual structural damage to the brain can cause a number of types of disorders, such as mental retardation and certain learning disorders. For example, degeneration of brain cells can cause dementia such as that found in Alzheimer's disease.

When a physician examines a patient and makes a diagnosis, he compares the patient's physical capabilities with national averages. For example, when you visit the ophthalmologist, she will use an eye chart to test your vision. A patient with 20/20 vision has normal eyesight—in other words, those with perfect eyesight can read a required line on the chart at 20 feet away. However, there are people who have eyesight that is better than 20/20. And there are also millions of people who have less than 20/20 vision and who need various visual aids, such as eyeglasses. There are many other ways in which physicians conduct these kinds of comparisons.

In the case of AD/HD, patients exhibit a range of behaviors that are outside of the normal, average range of behaviors. With AD/HD, problems with attention, impulsivity, and hyperactivity characterize the disorder. At present, it is believed that attention-deficit/hyperactivity disorder is caused by problems in the executive function areas of the brain and with the neurotransmitter dopamine.

I've seen attention-deficit/hyperactivity disorder listed as ADD, ADHD, and AD/HD. Which abbreviation is correct?

For the past hundred years, AD/HD has been known by many different titles. At first, physicians referred to those with AD/HD as suffering from "minimal brain dysfunction." After World War II, the term was changed to "hyperkinesis," a Latin word that means "superactive," and children with the disorder were referred to as hyperkinetic children. Then, in the 1980s, the American Psychiatric Association, in the third edition of *Diagnostic and Statistical Manual of Mental Disorders,* or *DSM-III,* changed the name to attention-deficit disorder, or ADD, for children and adults with attention problems. In 1987, in the *DSM-III-R* (the revised version), the term "ADHD" was added to include those with hyperactivity.

In the *DSM-IV* publication in 1994, the American Psychiatric Association recategorized the disorder into three subtypes: inattentive, hyperactive-impulsive, and a combined type. The abbreviation "AD/HD" means that the individual can have the "AD," or attention-deficit subtype; the "H," or hyperactive-impulsive subtype; or the "AD/H," or both attention-deficit and hyperactive-impulsive subtype. It is an "either, or, and both" identification. In other Western countries, the term "hyperkinetic disorder" is still used. In the United States, the terms ADD, ADHD, and AD/HD are often still used interchangeably.

Does AD/HD really exist?

When my children were first diagnosed, I wrestled with this question. Even though I was a teacher, even though I had taught hundreds of children over the years and had seen evidence of AD/HD firsthand, I pondered this question seriously. In my quest for answers about the disorder and in my attempt to help my girls, I read everything I could about AD/HD. I researched the history of the disorder. I reviewed studies on medications. I boggled my mind with medical summaries, charts, and statistics. Finally, after years of concern as a parent and thousands of hours reading books and medical journals and doing Internet research, I came to a conclusion that millions of other parents, physicians, scientists, and those with AD/HD had already decided. *Yes, I believe that AD/HD does exist.* Below is a list of important scientific statistics that might help you in your decision:

- AD/HD is one of the most common and serious conditions, affecting approximately 3 to 7 percent of children in the United States. Recent studies suggest that actual numbers may be much higher.
- According to AD/HD expert Dr. Joseph Biederman of Harvard Medical School, AD/HD is the number-one reason that children and adolescents visit mental health professionals.

- Studies from the National Institute of Mental Health show that when children with AD/HD are given stimulants such as Ritalin, Metadate, Concerta, and Adderall, their handwriting improves significantly.
- Numerous medical studies have shown that the use of stimulant medications causes significant and measurable improvements in AD/HD-related behaviors.
- Anatomic studies of the brain using magnetic resonance images (MRI) indicate smaller brain volumes in AD/HD patients than in control subjects.
- Studies conducted on twins show substantial evidence of a genetic link with AD/HD.
- Studies in molecular genetics have shown that genes regulating dopamine production and distribution are involved with AD/HD.
- In 2002, over one hundred top scientists from around the world released the "2002 International Consensus Statement on AD/HD": "As a matter of science, the notion that AD/HD does not exist is simply wrong. All of the major medical associations and government health agencies recognize AD/HD as a genuine disorder because the scientific evidence indicating it is so overwhelming."

Why is AD/HD so controversial?

There are three primary reasons why AD/HD is so controversial.

1. Existence of AD/HD

Some parents and professionals don't believe that AD/HD exists. They believe that the child is being lazy or a daydreamer or strong-willed. "He just isn't applying himself," they say. They believe that if the child would work harder, the problem would be solved. One high-level psychiatrist once gave me his opinion. According to him, AD/HD behaviors in children were a result of bad parenting. As a parent of two AD/HD children, I gulped when he told me this. All of us can be better parents, me included, but I don't believe that AD/HD behaviors are a result of parenting skills.

I have found that the number of people and organizations that recognize

AD/HD as an actual disorder are staggering. Just a few of the organizations that are involved with AD/HD include the American Academy of Child and Adolescent Psychiatry (AACAP), the American Academy of Neurology (AAN), the American Academy of Pediatrics, the American Medical Association (AMA), the American Psychiatric Association, Attention-Deficit Information Network (AD-IN), the Council for Exceptional Children, the Federation of Families for Children's Mental Health, the HEATH Resource Center, Job Accommodation Network (JAN), the Mayo Clinic, NAMI (formerly the National Alliance for the Mentally Ill), the National Association of Private Special Education Centers, the national Attention-Deficit Disorder Association (ADDA), the National Center for Gender Issues and ADHD, the National Information Center for Children and Youth with Disabilities, the National Institute of Mental Health, the National Resource Center on AD/HD, and the Parent Advocacy Coalition for Educational Rights (PACER).

2. Stigma of mental illness

For many years, having a mental illness was a real stigma in our society. The attitude about mental disorders has changed a great deal. Many parents and professional understand that AD/HD is a disorder in the brain. Having it doesn't mean that a child is insane, inferior, bad, or stupid. For some parents, however, the possible stigma of having a child with a mental disorder is too difficult to accept. For these parents, it is often easier or less emotionally painful to think of their child's behavior as something else.

3. Use of stimulant medications to treat AD/HD children

This is the most hotly debated issue around AD/HD. Some people say that we are making our children "high" by giving them stimulant medications. Other people argue that early stimulant medication use will turn a child into a drug addict. Some people say that the medications aren't safe and that we don't know the results of long-term use. Others believe that AD/HD can be cured with natural diets rather than the use of medication.

The use of stimulants to treat AD/HD in children is the most widely researched treatment in the mental disorder arena. Hundreds of studies have been conducted. Research has shown that 75 to 90 percent of children with AD/HD symptoms show moderate to significant improvement.

What areas of the brain are affected by AD/HD?

Research using neuroimaging techniques, such as the MRI, has shown that a significant number of AD/HD children have regions in their brains that are smaller than average. The regions of the brain that are different in size and structure in AD/HD children include the prefrontal cortex, the cerebellum, and the basal ganglia. In addition to certain regions of the brain being smaller, research has shown that the *total* brain size of these children is 5 percent smaller than children without AD/HD.

What areas of behavior and learning do these affected areas of the brain control?

When I began doing research in this area, it was like a lightbulb effect. I remember thinking, *Wow! Now this makes sense!* I hope this brief description helps you understand this complicated disorder too.

Certain areas of the brain control certain behaviors and functions. In those with AD/HD, abnormalities have been discovered in the basal ganglia, prefrontal cortex, and cerebellum. But what do these areas of the brain control?

- Basal ganglia—This area of the brain helps control attention levels, thought processes, and movement.
- Prefrontal cortex—In general, this section of the brain helps us analyze social behaviors and control impulsive behaviors. It helps us decide what to pay attention to and what to ignore.
- Dorsolateral prefrontal circuits—These areas of the brain control attention and short-term memory.
- Orbitomedial prefrontal circuits—These areas help our brain weed out distractions.

- Ventral frontal circuits—This area of the brain helps control and inhibit behaviors, as well as serving to control our emotions and corresponding behaviors.
- Cerebellum—The cerebellum is involved in higher thinking skills such as logic, time-management, and reasoning skills. The midline vermis of the cerebellum, in particular, one of the smaller areas of the brain in children with AD/HD, helps control and modulate the brain's dopamine levels, as well as controlling energy and locomotion levels.

Why can't scientists use neuroimaging to determine whether an individual has AD/HD?

When scientists compare brain volume and size between those with AD/HD and those without the disorder, they are comparing large groups of people. Although they have frequently observed a consistent link between brain size and AD/HD, the percentage is too small to be used on an individual basis. Just as some people have smaller feet than others do, a slightly smaller brain might be normal for that individual and does not necessarily indicate a diagnosis of AD/HD.

What is the connection between dopamine and AD/HD?

Dopamine is a neurotransmitter found in the brain. Neurotransmitters are released to tell your brain what to do. Dopamine, in particular, helps initiate and control movement, energy, and alertness. Scientists have discovered that children with AD/HD have dopamine levels in their right midbrains that are 48 percent higher than those of children without AD/HD. These findings suggest abnormalities in dopa decarboxylase activity and other problems with receptor and uptake transporters. In scientific circles, the belief that the neurotransmitter plays a major role in AD/HD is called the dopamine hypothesis.

What causes AD/HD?

There are numerous factors that could "cause" or bring about AD/HD in a child:

- AD/HD can be an inherited disorder. Researchers have discovered abnormalities on two specific genes of those with AD/HD—the dopamine transporter gene on chromosome 5 (DAT1) and the dopamine receptor gene on chromosome 11 (DRD4).
- AD/HD is thought by experts to be caused by smaller executive function areas in the brain as well as problems with the supply and distribution of the neurotransmitter dopamine in the central nervous system.
- Prenatal complications including low birth weight of the fetus, premature delivery, and lack of oxygen to the fetus are thought to be possible causes.
- Mothers who smoked during pregnancy might have put their children at risk.
- Exposure to high levels of lead, such as ingesting paint chips containing lead as a young child, is a possible cause.

Does genetics play a major role in the development of AD/HD?

Your son is tall and has dark brown eyes and a small dimple at the end of his nose. He has his uncle's towering height, his grandmother's beautiful eyes, his great-grandfather's dimple, and maybe your AD/HD.

AD/HD often runs in families. Studies have shown that genetics plays a strong role in the development of AD/HD. Approximately 10 to 35 percent of AD/HD children have a mother or father with the disorder. And if a parent has the disorder, there is a 35 to 50 percent chance that *one* of the children has AD/HD as well. Studies on twins have also shown that identical twins have a much higher chance of sharing the disorder than fraternal twins.

Genetic research on AD/HD has pinpointed abnormalities in the dopaminergic (dopamine) system. These include variations on the following genes:

- dopamine-transporter (DAT1) gene on chromosome 5
- dopamine-receptor (DRD4) gene on chromosome 11
- dopamine receptor (DRD2-5) gene
- dopa decarboxylase (DDC) gene
- dopamine beta-hydroxylase (DBH) gene
- monoamine oxidase A (MAOA) gene

However, even though a child has a genetic variation on one of the genes, it doesn't necessarily mean that the child will inherit AD/HD. Scientists believe that it could take more than one genetic factor. Others believe that something must trigger the disorder, such as a lack of oxygen during birth or an environmental toxin.

In addition, studies have found that if more than one child in a family has AD/HD, the disorder doesn't necessarily remain in the same subtype. For example, one child could have the hyperactivity/impulsive (HI) subtype and the other child could have the inattentive (I) subtype.

According to Drs. Ogdie, Macphie, Minassian, and Yang (among others) in their 2003 journal article, there is a definite link between AD/HD and three other chromosome regions—16p13, 17p11, and 5p13. When scientists do a genomewide scan, they compare and contrast gene similarities and differences between groups of people. What they are looking for is a linkage or similarities on particular chromosomes. In the analysis performed by Ogdie and his associates, they performed the first genomewide scan on those with AD/HD. They discovered that study participants who had abnormalities in chromosome regions 16p13, 17p11, and 5p13 also had AD/HD. Studies like these help pinpoint genetic markers for disease and disorders. (Of particular note, these three genes have also been high-lighted in playing a part in the disorder of autism. See page 13.)

Can bad parenting cause AD/HD?

Experts disagree about the role of parenting as a risk factor in develop-ing AD/HD. In a 1995 study, researchers found that parents of AD/HD children are often too controlling and intrusive in their children's lives. However, other studies suggest that parents of AD/HD children are more controlling and intrusive because they have to be. These experts suggest that parents are responding to their AD/HD child's behavior rather than causing it.

Can bad parenting cause AD/HD? In my opinion, no. AD/HD is caused by disorders in the executive function areas of the brain. But bad parenting can make the behavioral aspects of AD/HD worse—much worse—as well as increasing feelings of depression, anxiety, low self-esteem, and worthlessness in the AD/HD child.

Parenting an AD/HD child might be the most difficult thing you ever do. Often, you might feel exhausted and overwhelmed. But no matter what else you do in your life, nothing is as important as your job as a par-ent. Your role as advocate, teacher, and coach is the key to your AD/HD child's success.

Can other disorders be confused with AD/HD?

Yes. Just a few of these include the following:

- oppositional defiant disorder (ODD)
- conduct disorder (CD)
- generalized anxiety disorder (GAD)

- separation anxiety disorder
- obsessive-compulsive disorder (OCD)
- major depressive disorder
- bipolar disorder
- dysthymic disorder
- autistic disorder
- Asperger's disorder
- learning disabilities (LD)

Can other disorders go along with AD/HD? What are these disorders?

Yes, numerous other disorders often exist along with AD/HD. A 1999 National Institute of Mental Health (NIMH) study found that two-thirds of AD/HD children also have at least one comorbid, or coexisting, condition. According to NIMH, comorbidity occurs in most AD/HD children in the following percentages:

- 40 percent of children with oppositional defiant disorders (ODD) also have AD/HD
- 30 to 35 percent of children with language disorders also have AD/HD
- 21 to 90 percent of children with tic disorders also have AD/HD
- 20 to 25 percent of children with anxiety disorders also have AD/HD
- 15 to 25 percent of children with learning disabilities also have AD/HD
- 15 to 20 percent of children with conduct disorders also have AD/HD
- 15 to 20 percent of children with mood disorders also have AD/HD

Is AD/HD related to Asperger's disorder or autism?

Clinically speaking, the two disorders are very different. AD/HD is distinguished by problems with inattention, hyperactivity, and impulsivity. Autism and autism spectrum disorders such as Asperger's are characterized by social skill malfunctions and repetitious behaviors, such as rocking or spinning objects.

There does seem to be some overlap between the two disorders, however. Both AD/HD children and autistic children have problems in the social skill arena. Both disorders are also characterized by deficits in the executive function areas of the brain. Genomewide scans for AD/HD and autism have found three genetic markers for both disorders—16p13, 17p11, and 5p13.

Further research needs to be conducted to determine the significance of these symptom similarities and the importance of the shared genetic markers.

Is AD/HD caused by a food or chemical allergy?

There is no scientific evidence that AD/HD is caused by a food allergy, a chemical sensitivity, or the lack of something in the diet.

There will be some people who will disagree with me about food allergies. All scientific evidence to date points to the fact that people are born with AD/HD, although in a few cases the disorder has been caused by an accident with injury to the brain or by exposure to lead. AD/HD is caused by a problem in the brain and with the release and uptake of the neurostransmitter dopamine. If someone said he could improve your child's learning disabilities with diet, most of us would shake our heads, knowing it can't be done. If someone said he had a "cure" for cerebral palsy or mental retardation, many of us would be angry. But because AD/HD is caused by a chemical as well as a structural problem in the brain, some people say that what a child eats can resolve that problem. However, dopamine is not found in food or organic substances. It is a neurotransmitter that the brain produces.

Those who say they can cure the disorder by changing a child's diet are not telling you the truth, or they are making an assumption about something that hasn't been proven to work.

How common is AD/HD in children?

In the United States, approximately 3 to 7 percent of school-age children have been diagnosed with AD/HD. Some experts estimate that the number may be as high as 5 to 10 percent. Statistically, boys are two or three times more likely to have AD/HD than girls, and are also more likely to have the hyperactive/impulsive or the combined subtype. Girls often have the inattentive subtype. Caucasian children are two times more likely to be diagnosed with AD/HD than African-American or Hispanic children.

Here is another way to look at these numbers: Let's imagine that a grade school has four third-grade classes with twenty-five students in each class. If we take the smallest number that experts agree upon, 5 percent, then 5 students out of 100 will have AD/HD. This means that, on average, each class will have at least one AD/HD student.

Can a child grow out of AD/HD?

For many years, it was thought that children with AD/HD often "outgrow" the disorder. Now it is believed that AD/HD is a life span disorder, or a disorder that you have your whole life.

Can AD/HD be cured?

No, not at this time. Be careful of websites declaring guaranteed cures for AD/HD. Remember, experts believe that AD/HD is caused by problems in the right frontal lobe of the brain and with the distribution of the neurotransmitter dopamine. At this time there are no cures for the size and structure of a person's brain.

Has the number of people with AD/HD gone up in the past few years?

There are more people who have been diagnosed as having AD/HD. This doesn't necessarily mean that more people have AD/HD. Perhaps the increased numbers mean that we are more educated about the disorder and better at identifying it. But the increase *might* mean that more children do have AD/HD than in previous years. Studies need to be conducted to determine why the numbers are up.

How does AD/HD affect our society? How does it affect AD/HD children?

AD/HD is a serious health concern. The direct and indirect costs of the disorder are numerous, including the following:

- Children and adolescents with AD/HD have more accidents and incur higher medical costs than children without AD/HD. (Centers for Disease Control and Prevention)
- Although causation has not been clearly proven, AD/HD children are five times more likely to die from an accident than children without AD/HD.

- According to Medicaid figures, average treatments costs for AD/HD children, including the costs for their medications, is $1,795 per year. That is about $100 more than Medicaid costs for children with asthma per year.
- Experts now believe that AD/HD is not "outgrown" as previously believed, but that the disorder continues into adulthood. Adults with AD/HD have higher rates of mental health problems, unemployment, substance abuse issues, marital difficulties, and divorce rates, as well as higher rates of criminal activity and incarceration in correctional facilities than those without AD/HD.

As a parent of two AD/HD children, I am concerned about these statistics. Raising a child in today's society is a tremendous responsibility and a huge challenge. When you have a child with AD/HD, your job is even more difficult. But I do believe that there is hope for our AD/HD children. Helping your AD/HD child grow up to be a happy, productive adult will be one of the most difficult things you will ever do. But with a lot of love and patience, with education and coaching and medication, it can be done. Regardless of these discouraging statistics, there is hope for your AD/HD child too!

Why is it so important to treat AD/HD?

Correct diagnosis, including any comorbid conditions, and effective treatment programs, including medication, for AD/HD individuals are absolutely essential—for the happiness and well-being of our AD/HD children and the stability of our country. I believe that AD/HD is one of the most important mental health issues of this century. Below are just a few ways that untreated AD/HD can negatively effect our world:

- Lower academic performance level of children with AD/HD. Eighty to 90 percent are behind their peers by the sixth grade.
- Increased level of school suspensions experienced by AD/HD children. Up to 50 percent of AD/HD children receive school suspensions.

- Poor self-esteem and social difficulties.
- Increased risk of accidental injuries.
- Increased risk for automobile accidents and citations experienced by teens and adults with AD/HD.
- The premarital pregnancy rate in teenagers with AD/HD is nine times higher than that of their non-AD/HD peers.
- Higher divorce rates in families with an AD/HD child or adult. The divorce rate is more than twice as high when someone with AD/HD marries.
- High cost of education ($3.5 to $4 million) spent yearly for AD/HD children receiving special services.
- Adoption difficulties.
- Increased risk of substance abuse for teens and adults with AD/HD.
- Other social costs, including criminal activity, homelessness, and poverty.
- Adults with AD/HD are four to five times as likely to be fired from a job.
- High percentage of individuals with AD/HD in both the juvenile and adult justice systems.

2.

SYMPTOMS OF AD/HD

· ·

Children with AD/HD have numerous symptoms that characterize the disorder, such as inattention or hyperactivity. The difficulty is that many of these symptoms can also be found in other disorders. Is it AD/HD? Or is it conduct disorder or learning disabilities? Are your child's symptoms part of more than one disorder? Identifying the symptoms of AD/HD and correctly identifying the disorder and any coexisting disorders is one of the first steps in the treatment process.

What are the symptoms of AD/HD?

According to the American Psychiatric Association's *Diagnostic and Statistical Manual of Mental Disorders (DSM-IV)*, six or more of the symptoms listed below are necessary to receive a diagnosis of AD/HD. In addition, the symptoms must have existed for six months or more and be severe enough to be out of the normal range of development for the person's age group.

INATTENTION

- Often fails to give close attention to details or makes careless mistakes in schoolwork, work, or other activities.
- Often has difficulty sustaining attention in tasks or play activities.
- Often does not seem to listen when spoken to directly.
- Often does not follow through on instructions and fails to finish schoolwork, chores, or duties in the workplace (not due to oppositional behavior or failure to understand instructions).
- Often has difficulty organizing tasks and activities.
- Often avoids, dislikes, or is reluctant to engage in tasks that require sustained mental effort (such as schoolwork or homework).
- Often loses things necessary for tasks or activities (e.g., toys, school assignments, pencils, books, or tools).
- Is often easily distracted by extraneous stimuli.
- Is often forgetful in daily activities.

HYPERACTIVITY

- Often fidgets with hands or feet or squirms in seat.
- Often leaves seat in classroom or in other situations in which remaining seated is expected.
- Often runs about or climbs excessively in situations in which it is inappropriate (in adolescents or adults, may be limited to subjective feelings of restlessness).
- Often has difficulty playing or engaging in leisure activities quietly.
- Is often "on the go" or often acts as if "driven by a motor."
- Often talks excessively.

IMPULSIVITY

- Often blurts out answers before questions have been completed.
- Often has difficulty awaiting turn.
- Often interrupts or intrudes on others (e.g., butts into conversations or games).
- Some hyperactive-impulsive or inattentive symptoms that cause impairment were present before age seven years.
- Some impairment from the symptoms is present in two or more settings (e.g., at school [or work] and at home).

- There must be clear evidence of clinically significant impairment in social, academic, or occupational functioning.
- The symptoms do not occur exclusively during the course of a pervasive developmental disorder, schizophrenia, or other psychotic disorder and are not better accounted for by another mental disorder (e.g., mood disorder, anxiety disorder, dissociative disorder, or a personality disorder).

Reprinted with permission from the *Diagnostic and Statistical Manual of Mental Disorders,* Copyright © 2000 American Psychiatric Association.

Approximately 75 percent of patients who have been diagnosed with AD/HD have the combined type, with inattention, hyperactivity, and impulsivity. Fifteen to 20 percent have the inattention subtype, while the remaining 5 percent have hyperactivity and impulsivity symptoms but not problems with inattention.

Do children with AD/HD sometimes have sensory problems?

Yes. Children with AD/HD are sometimes overly sensitive to sound and touch. Loud noises or music can cause an AD/HD child to cover his ears or to run out of the room. Loud volumes, such as those found in movie theaters or concerts, can cause an AD/HD child with sensory problems to become frightened or upset.

Children with AD/HD and children with other disorders as well can have difficulties in three sensory areas—tactile or touch, proprioceptive or spatial relationships, and vestibular or balanced movement.

Tactile difficulties are sometimes also tactile defensiveness. Children who have problems in this area often don't like things touching them. This can include certain types or materials of clothing, buttons, snaps, zippers, elastic, and manufacturer tags. It can include aversions to getting their hair cut or taking baths. Children who are tactile-defensive sometimes don't like messy play—such as getting their hands in clay, paint, or Play-Doh.

The second sensory area is proprioceptive. The proprioceptive system, which relates to the position of the body in space, allows us to know what our body parts are doing, how fast or slow we need to move, and how much pressure to use. Children with difficulties in this sensory area often appear clumsy and uncoordinated or can appear stiff in their movements. These children often throw the ball too fast, hug too hard, and cause cats and dogs and sometimes peers to hide. If this sensory area is not treated, these children can sometimes grow up thinking, "I'm terrible at sports" or "No one likes me."

When I was growing up, my mother developed a program for my autistic brother, Scott. One of the activities involved proprioceptive issues. I remember a "hugging" exercise. I would tell Scott to give me a hug. I remember saying many times, "Oo, too hard, Scott. Too hard! Not so tight!" Every day, each person in the family had a series of 15-minute lessons or exercises with Scott. These exercises were repeated many, many times over the years. The program that my mother developed for my brother is the main catalyst behind the coaching program and exercises in Chapter 10 (see pages 109ff).

The third sensory issue is vestibular. The vestibular, or balanced movement, system provides our brain with information about our environment. It tells us where we are in space—for example, sitting or crouching. It is also involved with right/left movements and balance. The vestibular system moves our eyes and head and allows us to know which hand to use. Children with vestibular problems are typically clumsy in their movements. They might fall often, tip over chairs, and trip over items.

These sensory processing problems can be a result of abnormalities in the cerebellum. If your child has sensory difficulties, an occupational therapist can help analyze his or her needs and establish a sensory integration program. Below are just a few of the calming strategies used to help a child with sensory issues:

- rocking chairs and swings
- weighted vests
- fidgets or stress balls
- padded chairs
- Wilbarger Protocol for Deep Touch Pressure
- deep pressure massage

- warm baths
- chewing gum or ice

In Chapter 10, there are exercises to help your child cope with tactile difficulties.

For further information on sensory processing problems, please see the following sources:

- Belle Curve Records, Inc. at (888) 357-5867
  or http://www.sensoryresources.com
- Sensory Integration International at (310) 320-9986
  or http://home.earthlink.net/~sensoryint/
- The SPD Network at http://www.sinetwork.org
- Sensory Comfort at http://www.sensorycomfort.com
- *The Out-of-Sync Child,* by Carol Stock Kranowitz

What other behaviors do children with AD/HD display?

Children with AD/HD can display a host of other behaviors. Often these behaviors exist because of coexisting, or comorbid, disorders, such as various conduct or mood disorders. A few other behaviors that can go along with AD/HD include:

- temper tantrums or meltdowns
- angry outbursts
- hysteria over the loss or misplacement of a toy or other item
- aggression toward siblings or peers
- depression or sadness
- disregard of safety issues
- apparent lack of "common sense" in a situation (for example, climbing on a high object even after they have fallen off and gotten hurt previously)

- sensory problems such as auditory sensitivities and tactile defensiveness
- difficulty in maintaining good hygiene
- poor short-term and long-term memory—including often forgetting assignments, textbooks, and instructions
- inconsistent behaviors
- frequent loss or misplacement of items
- inapppropriate noises
- loud speaking voice
- invasion of personal space, such as getting right in people's faces when talking
- touching or grabbing other people in inappropriate ways or at inappropriate times
- submissive behaviors
- constantly asking for things
- failure to complete tasks
- immature behavior below their age level
- overly sensitive; experiencing hurt feelings with little or no provocation
- easily frustrated with failure or difficult tasks
- uncooperative and defiant behavior with parents and/or teachers
- failure to follow or understand social cues or rules
- sudden and rapid mood changes
- refusal to accept responsibility for mistakes

Could temper tantrums and fits be a symptom of AD/HD?

Temper tantrums, fits, or meltdowns, as they are sometimes called, can have numerous causes:

- Studies have shown that AD/HD children and also adults with AD/HD have greater emotional lability problems than the average person.
- Some of the medications used to treat AD/HD can heighten these issues in some children.

- Frequent meltdowns in an AD/HD child can be a sign of a comorbid disorders such as conduct disorder, Asperger's disorder, or depression.
- Medications used to treat comorbid disorders can sometimes cause temper outbursts and crying jags.
- When the stimulant medications are wearing off, some AD/HD children will have a meltdown as a result.

AD/HD meltdowns are often more intense and longer than a temper tantrum that an average child might have over a lost toy or privilege. If your child is having a problem with meltdowns, you need to be a detective of sorts, to help your child. For a couple of weeks, keep a record of the meltdowns. Record how long each meltdown lasted, the time of day, and the cause or trigger, if it can be identified. When you meet with your AD/HD specialist to discuss the meltdowns, bring your list. By keeping accurate records of the behavior, you might be able to see a pattern. Here are two examples:

EXAMPLE 1			
Monday	10 minutes	5:10–5:20 p.m.	Homework
Tuesday	15 minutes	5:30–5:45 p.m.	Favorite TV show wasn't on
	30 minutes	9:30–10:00 p.m.	Refused to go to bed
Wednesday	12 minutes	5:00–5:12 p.m.	Refused to do homework (went to bed early)
Thursday	None		
Friday	5 minutes	4:55–5:00 p.m.	Lost favorite toy

Notice a couple of patterns with this example. First of all, most of the meltdowns seem to be occurring around 5 p.m. Perhaps the child is on a medication that is wearing off. A possible solution would be to try a longer lasting medication or take a small "booster" pill at 4 p.m. Also, notice that there were no meltdowns on Thursday. This might mean that the child is not getting enough sleep.

EXAMPLE 2			
Monday	5 minutes	4:30–4:35 p.m.	Refused to do homework
Tuesday	10 minutes	7:30–7:40 a.m.	Got up early to do home-work from previous day. Cried.
Wednesday	30 minutes	7:00–7:30 a.m.	Cried. Said she hated school.
	45 minutes	4:00–4:45 p.m.	Fell on the ground kick ing. Didn't want to do homework.
Thursday	20 minutes	7:00–7:20 p.m.	Screamed, saying school was unfair.
Friday	None		

Do you notice a pattern here? The problem seems to be an aversion to school. In this case, the child might be having problems with peers and feel rejected. Or the child might have a learning disability and might be having a very difficult time doing the assignment projects. Obviously, the child is feeling very frustrated and anxious about school.

I treat meltdowns as if the child were having a seizure. When one is coming on, move the child to a quiet place and wait. Just as getting mad at a child for having a seizure wouldn't help and would actually be cruel and thoughtless, it doesn't help with an AD/HD meltdown either. Don't try to talk or reason with your child until after the meltdown is over. Try to find techniques that can help, such as a deep pressure hug. When the meltdown is over, say the following: "Are you okay now? Is there anything you need? (For example, a cool drink or a nap.) What do you think triggered your meltdown? If this happens again, what are some other options to help you stay in control?"

If your child is having AD/HD meltdowns, it is essential that you work with your AD/HD specialist to find out the cause. When you notice patterns and triggers, you can begin to treat the problem.

STEPS TO TAKE WHEN YOUR CHILD
IS HAVING A MELTDOWN
. . . . . .

Stay calm.

Don't get angry.

Don't yell or spank the child.

Don't say much. When you do, talk in quiet, calm tones.

If you are in a public place, try to move the child to a quieter, more private location.

Don't try to question the child while the meltdown is taking place.

Do say, "Shh, it's okay. You're all right."

If the child likes deep pressure touch, hold the child securely in your arms.

After the meltdown is over, say, "Are you okay now? Is there anything you need?" (Like a glass of water or a nap)

Talk about what options he or she has in the future to avoid having a meltdown.

Give the child a hug. Say, "I love you."

Do vocal and physical tics sometimes go along with AD/HD?

Yes. According to a news release from the American Academy of Neurology, 90 percent of those with tic disorders also have AD/HD. In addition, some of the medications used to treat AD/HD can worsen or bring out latent tic disorders. What does this mean? It means that the stimulant medications can sometimes magnify or increase vocal and physical tics. In other words, your child might have had a very small tic disorder before using the medications—so small that no one noticed. But after using stimulant medications for AD/HD, the disorder becomes more pronounced. For this reason, stimulant medications should be used with caution for children. Atomoxetine is a consideration to treat AD/HD in children with tic disorders.

Keep in mind also that it might not be the medication that is causing the problem. It could be the dosage level or the drug-release mechanism used (for example, extended-release rather than a short-acting tablet).

If your child has tic disorders or you notice a development of new tics after starting medication, talk to your AD/HD specialist.

Is there a higher occurrence of AD/HD in children with seizures?

Yes. About 20 to 35 percent of epileptic children also have AD/HD.

Do children with AD/HD experience sleep disorders?

Yes, studies have shown that numerous children with AD/HD have problems with sleep. This includes difficulties going to sleep quickly, difficulties staying asleep, and less time spent in sleep per night. Children with AD/HD and sleep disturbances should be evaluated for sleep-disordered breathing problems. Stimulants can cause sleep difficulties too. If your child is experiencing new sleep difficulties after being treated with a stimulant, you should discuss with your physician possibly lowering the dosage, changing the time of the dosage, or trying a different medication.

3.

DIAGNOSIS AND TESTS

. . . .

In many ways, attention-deficit/hyperactivity disorder is an ongoing diagnostic process. In the case of my children, an AD/HD specialist at a mental health facility tested Theresa when she was four. Before we put her on medication, she went through a series of evaluations and meetings with a different psychologist for two months. We then received a second diagnosis from the psychologist. When she started school, both the school and a new child psychiatrist evaluated her again. All four different evaluations pointed strongly toward an AD/HD diagnosis. When she was eight, she was diagnosed with obsessive-compulsive behavior. When she was ten, Asperger's disorder was added to the diagnosis. She is now ten. Dr. Van Haren diagnosed Jenny when she was in first grade. She was also put through a battery of tests by the school system, which diagnosed a learning disability in reading. Four times a year, we meet with Dr. Van Haren to discuss how things are going and how the medications are working.

As you can see, testing for AD/HD isn't fast or easy. This chapter will help answer any questions that you might have about the process.

How early can a child be tested for AD/HD?

There are numerous difficulties and factors to consider when testing a child younger than six for AD/HD. First of all, the *DSM-IV* classification system, the standard criteria used from the American Psychiatric Association's *Diagnostic and Statistical Manual IV*, was not designed for use with children younger than six. Preschool children can also exhibit AD/HD–type behaviors, such as hyperactivity or short attention spans, that might be normal for their age. Other preschoolers with AD/HD could possibly behave differently in a doctor's office, such as being quiet and timid in a new situation, and the disorder might not be picked up by the physician.

Of course testing a child may lead to another key question: "Should we treat AD/HD preschoolers with stimulants?"

There are difficulties with not putting a preschooler on medication. Studies have shown that AD/HD children as young as four can be excluded from play with their peers. Dextroamphetamine and amphetamine salts have been approved for children as young as three, while methylphenidate and atomoxetine have been approved for children over six.

But each child is different. I believe it depends on the level of severity of the disorder and the context in which the medication is used. If you believe your child has AD/HD, it doesn't hurt to have him tested at an early age. I would again have him retested a second and even a third time when he reaches school age. I believe that medication should be used on preschoolers only in extreme cases of hyperactivity and after a second opinion. In addition, children with AD/HD should also be evaluated for comorbid or coexisting disorders.

What is the best way to have my child tested for AD/HD?

If you or your school believes that your child has AD/HD, there are particular steps you should take in having your child tested. These include the following:

- Your pediatrician should conduct a complete evaluation of your child to rule out any other physical possibilities. Hearing and vision should be checked.
- After the physical, ask your pediatrician to recommend a child psychologist or psychiatrist in your area who specializes in diagnosing and treating AD/HD.
- Meet with the specialist to talk about your child.
- The specialist should use criteria from the American Psychiatric Association's *Diagnostic and Statistical Manual (DSM-IV)* to evaluate your child. In other Western countries, the World Health Organization's *International Classification of Diseases (ICD-10)* is used to diagnose hyperkinetic disorder (HKD)—the WHO term for AD/HD.
- Both the parents and the school system should be involved in the diagnose process. Often parents are asked to fill out the Conners' Parent Rating Scale, while teachers complete the Conners' Teacher Rating Scale.
- The specialist should meet with the child for at least three visits to complete the evaluation. It is optimal to meet for more than three sessions—often up to six.
- The specialist should also evaluate the child for comorbid disorders, such as learning disabilities, Asperger's disorder, and oppositional-defiant disorders, among others.
- School systems also often test for learning disorders of various types. Ask to have your child evaluated.
- When your child is first diagnosed, you should meet with the AD/HD specialist often—once a week until the medication dosage is sta-

bilized. After your specialist has determined the best medication and dosage for your child, you and your child should meet with the AD/ HD specialist on a quarterly basis. You should bring copies of report cards, notes from teachers, and some copies of homework and artwork. Don't just focus on the negative—show examples of a "job well done" too. Be prepared to discuss any problems that your child is having, as well as talking about how the child is doing on his current medication.

Besides the *DSM-IV,* what other tests are used to evaluate a child for AD/HD?

As I mentioned, guidelines from the *DSM-IV* are the general standard used, as well as Conners' Parent and Teacher Rating Scales. Other tests are used to look for symptoms of AD/HD, as well as testing intelligence levels, screening for behavioral and mood disorders, and comorbid disorders. Just a few of the other tests sometimes used include the following:

OTHER TESTS USED WHEN EVALUATING A CHILD FOR AD/HD:

Parent-completed AD/HD questionnaires
- Barkley Home Situations Questionnaire
- Child Behavior Checklist (CBCL) (Achenbach and Edelbrock)
- Conners' Parent Rating Scale
- Home Situations Questionnaire—Revised (HSQ-R)
- Iowa Conners' Parent Rating Scale
- The Scale of Behavioral Problems (Navarro, Peiro, Llacer, and Silva)

Teacher-completed AD/HD questionnaires
- Academic Performance Rating Scale (APRS)
- Child Behavior Checklist, Teacher Report Form (Achenbach and Edelbrock)
- Comprehensive Teacher Rating Scale (ACTeRS)
- Conners' Teacher Rating Scale
- Iowa Conners' Teacher Rating Scale—Based on the Conners'

Teacher Rating Scale, this teacher report form compares AD/HD-type behavior with oppositional-defiant behavior
- Self-Control Rating Scale (Kendall and Wilcox, 1979)
- School Problem Inventory (Miranda, Martorell, Llacer, Peiro, and Silva, 1993)
- Teacher Rating of Academic Achievement Motivation (TRAAM)

Parent- or teacher-completed AD/HD questionnaires
- Burks' Behavior Rating Scales, selected subscales
- Conners' Rating Scale (unspecified)
- SKAMP (a 10-item scale that measures how well a child functions at school and at home)
- SNAP-IV (a 26-item scale is based on the *DSM-IV* criteria)

Laboratory measures of AD/HD symptoms
- Children's Depression Inventory (CDI) (a test that looks for abnormal amounts of sadness or depression in a child)
- Conners' Continuous Performance Test
- Diagnostic Interview Schedule for Children (DISC) (used to assess mood disorders in children)
- Freedom from Distractibility Factor V (WISC-R and WISC-III)
- How I Feel About School Scale (HIFAS)
- Kagan Matching Familiar Figures Test
- Lindgren Continuous Performance Test
- Margolis Children's Checking Task
- Revised Children's Manifest Anxiety Scale (R-CMAS) (used to assess anxiety levels in children)
- Test of Variables of Attention
- Wechsler Intelligence Scale for Children, Revised (WISC-R) (a scale that tests intelligence levels against ability levels)

Why does the physician look for signs of coexisting disorders in a child with AD/HD?

A doctor looks for other coexisting, or comorbid, disorders for two reasons. Sometimes a child is misdiagnosed with AD/HD when the actual problem is something else, such as oppositional-defiant disorder or learning disabilities. Another reason she looks for other disorders in your AD/HD child is that other disorders often coexist with AD/HD. When a doctor is reviewing your child's evaluation, she is looking for errors in the diagnosis as well as the existence of comorbid disorders.

Is the school involved in testing?

Yes, they should be. The Individuals with Disabilities Education Act (IDEA) mandates that public education supply appropriate services to children with disabilities. If your child is suspected of having a disability that limits his ability to function in an academic setting, testing is required. This policy applies to children ages three to twenty-one. Under IDEA, AD/HD is listed as a condition that qualifies for special education services. If the school does not perform adequate testing of the child, parents can ask for an evaluation by another specialist at the school's expense. If your child qualifies, an individualized education plan (known by school officials as an IEP) will be designed for your AD/HD child by the school system. Numerous individuals are involved in this process, including parents, teachers, special education teachers, the school psychologist or social worker, and the principal. All of these rights for children with AD/HD are guaranteed by the IDEA.

What can I expect during testing? How long will it take?

You should expect the following during testing of your child:

- There should be an initial visit with your pediatrician.
- There should be at least three visits with the recommended AD/HD specialist. These visits can last one or more hours.
- You and your significant other will be asked to fill out numerous questionnaires, as both parents' opinions are often accessed.
- Your child's teacher will also be asked to fill out questionnaires.
- There will be possible additional testing by your child's school for AD/HD and other learning-related disorders.
- If your child is determined to have AD/HD, your school or you may request an individualized education program, which could involve more testing and meetings with involved school personnel.
- There should be other testing by your school and AD/HD specialist to determine if any comorbid conditions exist along with the AD/HD.

All of these tests could take up to two months or more. Also, keep in mind that it can sometimes take more than two months before you can finally get in to see a doctor, especially ones who are in special fields.

Should we get a second opinion?

Absolutely. Even if you trust the opinion of your first doctor, second opinions in this case are wise. The diagnosis will last a lifetime. You need to be sure that it is accurate and not made hastily. I particularly recommend a second or third opinion if your child is very young when first diagnosed.

What will happen after my child receives an AD/HD diagnosis?

In most cases, medication will be prescribed. Sometimes more than one medication will need to be tried before a "winner" is found. You, your AD/HD specialist, and your child's school should also develop a multimodal management plan for treatment. This plan can include counseling, behavior management plans, and coaching (see Chapters 9 and 10).

Can my child be mistakenly diagnosed with AD/HD?

Yes, your child can be given an incorrect diagnosis of AD/HD. There are no blood tests or any other definitive tests for the disorder. Therefore, it is extremely important that the diagnosis is done carefully. A diagnosis should be attained only after multiple visits and a thorough evaluation.

Is AD/HD overdiagnosed or underdiagnosed?

The parameters for diagnosing the disorder at this time are not completely clear. For example, what tests should be used? How many visits with the professional should a child have? How many people should be involved in the diagnostic process? Is the school involved? Incongruities in the answers to these questions create numerous problems. When a diagnosis is made too quickly, children who have behavioral and emotional problems can be incorrectly diagnosed with AD/HD. Sometimes a child is diagnosed as a very young child. In these cases, normal behaviors that resemble AD/HD can be mistaken for the disorder. Sometimes parents and schools are too quick to want a solution. Mistakes can be made out of desperation and inadequate or incomplete assessments.

But sometimes diagnoses can also be overlooked. There are many reasons why some children with AD/HD are not diagnosed, including the following:

- Some families do not have insurance and cannot afford the high costs of health care, including the cost of the diagnostic process.
- Most of the costs of mental health care are not covered by public aid programs.
- Some insurance plans do not cover mental health services, including the evaluation and treatment of AD/HD.
- Some insurance plans have high out-of-pocket costs for medications not available in a generic form.
- AD/HD may not be impairing enough for some children to be listed as a special education disorder, and therefore schools will not receive special funding for such children. Because of this, numerous children do not receive the assistance that they need, especially in low-income school districts.
- Minority children with AD/HD, and children from low-income areas, experience numerous barriers to diagnosis and treatment.
- Concern about medication risks may cause parents to resist seeking treatment for their child.
- There is a belief by some individuals that the disorder does not exist.
- There is a belief by some parents that the symptoms of AD/HD are caused by having a defiant, willful, or lazy child.
- There is fear by families that their child will be stigmatized if labeled with AD/HD.
- There is concern and embarrassment by families about taking their child to a mental health professional.
- There may be concern by parents that the real reason their child acts the way he does is because they are poor parents.
- The symptoms of AD/HD can be confused for other disorders and incorrectly diagnosed.

Q Our daughter is in high school and was just diagnosed with AD/HD. How could we have missed it for this long?

Sometimes it is obvious when someone has a disorder. Sometimes it is not. In addition, there are numerous other issues that can make getting a diagnosis, and a *correct* diagnosis, even more difficult. Children with the inattentive subtype of AD/HD often are more difficult to diagnose than the hyperactive-impulsive and combined subtypes. Inattentive-subtype children are often labeled as daydreamers. They are sometimes quiet and shy. Because they are not "in someone's face" all the time, their disorder can easily be overlooked or misconstrued as something else. With both the hyperactive/impulsive and the combined type, the child's behavior is often more obvious. Children in this subtype tend to have more behavior problems. They get in trouble at school and tease siblings. They talk nonstop and speak out of turn. They act impulsively and sometimes do things that are a danger to themselves or others. These high-visibility behaviors are usually what bring about a visit to the child psychiatrist or pediatrician for evaluation.

Another issue that makes diagnosis difficult is the different levels or severities of the disorder. Within the three subtypes, there are wide ranges on how hyperactive, impulsive, or inattentive someone is. In one case, a child might be slightly hyperactive, needing less sleep than others and constantly on the go. At first, parents and teachers might think that he is a "high-energy kid." In another case, a child might be literally leaping over the furniture—head first!

Additionally, other disorders often go along with AD/HD. Whew! Isn't one disorder enough? When more than one disorder exist together, they are called comorbidities. Just a few of the possible comorbidities are tic disorders, obsessive-compulsive disorders, dyslexia, Asperger's disorder, and numerous behavior disorders. When an individual has more than one disorder, it makes getting a "correct" diagnosis much more difficult.

Finally, there are no physical tests for AD/HD. In other words, there are no blood tests or other medical tests that can be given to a patient to pinpoint AD/HD. There have been some exciting new discoveries made recently, which might someday make diagnosing AD/HD a little easier. In 2003, scientists discovered that AD/HD patients have regions of their brains that are smaller in size—in particular, the prefrontal cortex, basal ganglia, and cerebellum regions of the brain. Because this discovery is so very new, scientists have not yet learned how to apply those discoveries to the actual diagnostic process. Perhaps one day in the future, scientists will be able to use magnetic resonance imaging and other yet unknown scientific tools to help in the process.

4.

MEDICATION

. . . .

Should we use medication to treat our child's AD/HD? Is it safe? Will it make a difference? All parents with an AD/HD child sooner or later must search for an answer to these questions. In my quest to help my two girls, I have done a complete reversal in my thinking. I hope that the answers to these questions help you too in making your decision.

What medications are used to help someone with AD/HD cope with his or her disorder?

Both stimulants and selective norepinephrine reputake inhibitors (SNRI) are used to help treat AD/HD. Below is a chart with information on the medications often prescribed:

BRAND NAME	RITALIN	METADATE
Generic name	methylphenidate	methylphenidate
Marketed by	Novartis Pharmaceuticals Corp.	Celltech
How it works	Central nervous system (CNS) stimulant	Central nervous system (CNS) stimulant
Type of pill	Immediate-release tablet, extended-release tablet (SR), or extended-release capsule (LA)	Intermediate-acting extended-release tablet and long-acting, extended-release capsule (CD)
Pill sizes	Ritalin tablet 5, 10, 20 mg; Ritalin sustained-release (SR) tablet 20 mg; Ritalin extended-release capsule 10, 20, 30, and 40 mg	10 and 20 mg extended-release tablet (Metadate ER); 10, 20, and 30 mg extended-release capsule (Metadate CD)
How it's taken	Tablet swallowed intact; Capsule swallowed intact or opened and sprinkled in applesauce	Swallowed intact or opened and sprinkled in applesauce
Recommended for age	6 and up	6 and up
How long it lasts	Short-acting tablet, 3–4 hours; sustained-release tablet or capsule, 6–8 hours	12 hours

CONCERTA	ADDERALL	DEXEDRINE	STRATTERA
methylphenidate	amphetamine salts	dextroamphetamine	atomoxetine
McNeil Consumer & Specialty Pharmaceuticals	Shire US Inc.	GlaxoSmithKline	Eli Lilly and Company
Central nervous system (CNS) stimulant	Central nervous system (CNS) stimulant	Central nervous system (CNS) stimulant	Selective norepinephrine reuptake inhibitors (SNRIs)
Extended-release tablet	Intermediate-acting extended-release capsule	Short-acting tablet or long-acting, extended-release capsule (spansule)	Capsule
18, 27, 36, and 54 mg extended-release tablet	5, 10, 15, 20, 25, and 30 mg extended-release capsule	5 mg tablet; 5, 10, and 15 mg (Dexedrine spansule) extended-release capsule	10, 18, 25, 40, and 60 mg capsule
Swallowed intact	Swallowed intact or opened and sprinkled in applesauce	Swallowed intact	Swallowed intact
6 and up	3 and up	3 and up	6 and up
6–8 hours	3–4 hours	short-acting tablet, 3–4 hours; spansule, 6–8 hours	3–4 hours

BRAND NAME	RITALIN	METADATE
Possible side effects	Decreased appetite, insomnia, irritability, headache, increase of tics	Decreased appetite, insomnia, irritability, headache, increase of tics
Rare side effects	Nausea, vomiting, dizziness, nervousness, tics, allergic reactions, increased blood pressure, and psychosis	Nausea, vomiting, dizziness, nervousness, tics, allergic reactions, increased blood pressure, and psychosis
Should not be used by	Those with significant anxiety, tension, and agitation; glaucoma; tics or Tourette's syndrome; current/recent use of an MAOI; patients with allergies to methylphenidate or any of the other ingredients in Ritalin	Those with significant anxiety, tension, and agitation; glaucoma; tics or Tourette's syndrome; current/recent use of an MAOI; patients with allergies to methylphenidate or any of the other ingredients in Metadate

CONCERTA	ADDERALL	DEXEDRINE	STRATTERA
Headache, stomach pain, sleeplessness, decreased appetite	Decreased appetite, insomnia, irritability, nausea, headache, increase of tics	Decreased appetite, insomnia, irritability, nausea, headache, increase of tics	Dyspepsia, nausea, vomiting, fatigue, decreased appetite, dizziness, mood swings
Nausea, vomiting, dizziness, nervousness, tics, allergic reactions, increased blood pressure, and psychosis	Blood pressure changes (higher in African-Americans), euphoria, hallucinations, and sudden death	Blood pressure changes (higher in African-Americans), euphoria, hallucinations	Allergic reactions including angioneurotic edema, urticaria, rash, and blood pressure changes
Those with significant anxiety, tension, and agitation; glaucoma; tics or Tourette's syndrome; current/recent use of an MAOI; patients with allergies to methylphenidate or any of the other ingredients in Concerta	Those with marked anxiety, tension and agitation; glaucoma; tics or Tourette's syndrome; anyone taking an MAOI; anyone with a history of drug abuse	Those with marked anxiety, tension and agitation; glaucoma; tics or Tourette's syndrome; anyone taking an MAOI; anyone with a history of drug abuse	Those with glaucoma, anyone taking an MAOI, patients with allergies to atomoxetine

BRAND NAME	RITALIN	METADATE
Websites for information	www.adhdinfo.com	www.metadate-cd.com
Phone numbers for information	888-669-6682	888-METADATE
Special notes	Do not take after 6 p.m.	Do not take after 6 p.m.

How do these medications work? Are they helpful?

Central nervous system (CNS) stimulant medications (such as Ritalin, Dexedrine, Metadate, Concerta, and Adderall) and nonstimulant medications (selective norepinephrine reputake inhibitor medication, Strattera) work by interacting with dopamine, serotonin, and norepinephrine transporters. These medications are mimics. They interact with neurotransporters that our brains produce. Ritalin, Metadate, Concerta, Dexedrine, and Adderall work by increasing the amounts of dopamine and norepinephrine to the brain. SNRIs (Strattera) work by blocking norepinephrine transporters only. The exact process by which these medications work is not completely understood.

ONCERTA	ADDERALL	DEXEDRINE	STRATTERA
ww.Concerta.net r www.focuson dhd.com	www.ADDER ALL-XR.com or www.adhdsupport company.com	www.gsk.com	www.strattera.com
88-440-7903	800-536-7878	888-825-5249	800-LILLY-RX
ake once aily in the norning, wallowed vhole and not hewed or rushed.	Do not take after 6 p.m.	Do not take after 6 p.m. Contains Yellow No. 5 food coloring (tartazine), which can cause severe allergic reactions in some people.	In very rare cases has been associated with liver injury

Approximately 75 to 90 percent of AD/HD children respond to stimulant treatment. If one medication doesn't work, try a different one. Statistics show that if one drug fails, there is a 25 percent chance another drug will have positive results.

Methylphenidate, dextroamphetamine, and amphetamine salt medications work quickly (within two days). Atomoxetine can take a month or more for results. These medications work by decreasing hyperactivity, impulsiveness, and emotional lability (inability to control emotions such as crying fits and temper tantrums). They also increase attention and short-term memory. Basically, these medications help AD/HD children to exhibit more "normal" behaviors. In addition, studies with AD/HD children have shown clear improvements in handwriting legibility while on medication.

In our family's experience, the transformation caused by the medications was incredible. It took a while before we got everything worked out. We had to try numerous medications and doses before we found something that worked. Even now, we sometimes have to tweak the medications. But the results were amazing. Within one week, Jenny jumped six reading levels. Theresa's handwriting became legible and she had fewer tantrums or meltdowns (only one or two a week, in comparison with three or four a day). We could sit at the dinner table and actually have a conversation. When a problem would occur, in most cases, we could sit down and discuss it, calmly and rationally. Everyone noticed the difference— teachers, grandparents, and neighbors.

For me, the big difference was seeing how the medication improved Theresa's handwriting. There is the saying "Seeing is believing." Seeing the changes the meds brought about in her writing made a believer of me. As a visual reference for you, I have included a sample of her handwriting taken 10 minutes before taking her medication, and then 30 minutes after taking her stimulant medication.

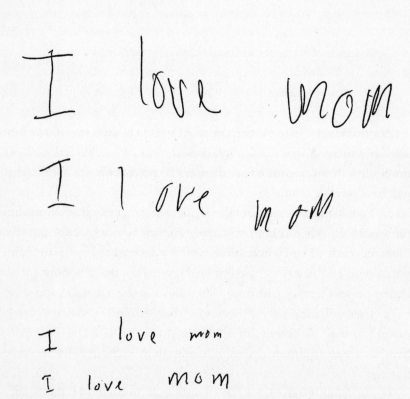

Are these medications like cocaine?

Methylphenidate, dextroamphetamine, and amphetamine salts are all stimulant medications. Nicotine and caffeine have some stimulant effects. Cocaine is a stimulant too. The medications used to treat AD/HD work by blocking the reuptake of dopamine and norepinephrine. The pill form of methylphenidate does not usually produce a "high" sensation, and studies have shown that it is not addictive when used appropriately. Cocaine, however, is a potent reuptake inhibitor. It works by blocking the reuptake of dopamine, norepinephrine, and serotonin as well.

Studies have shown that people with AD/HD have more dopamine transporters than those without AD/HD. This means that dopamine is being removed from their system faster than normal. In other words, the brain circuitry of those with AD/HD is being underfed. Stimulants work by supplying more dopamine to the system. SNRIs work by blocking the reuptake of norepinephrine, thereby allowing it to stay in the system longer.

Although methylphenidate, dextroamphetamine, amphetamine salts, and cocaine are all stimulants, they differ in a significant way. Medications for AD/HD are slow-acting. It takes about an hour for one of these drugs to increase the dopamine levels in the brain. Cocaine is different. When inhaled or injected, cocaine targets the brain in just seconds. How quickly the dopamine increases is key to the addiction process. Having said this, however, stimulant medications do have the potential to be abused. When injected as a liquid, it can produce a high and is in demand by drug addicts. This is why it is a controlled substance. Studies have shown that children who use stimulants to treat their AD/HD are less likely than their nonmedicated AD/HD counterparts to abuse drugs.

Are these medications safe?

As with any controversial issue, there are pros and cons to both sides. The drugs can create problems with appetite and sleep. Studies have shown that the stimulants do not measurably affect height, but they can affect weight. If stimulants are prescribed, careful monitoring of diet is important. Additionally, longer-lasting time-release medication may also interfere with normal sleep patterns. Despite these concerns, or perhaps because of them, the treatment of AD/HD in children with stimulants is one of the most widely researched treatments in the world. There have been literally hundreds of trials involving methylphenidate, amphetamine salts, and dextro-amphetamine. I am going to do my best to present both sides of this issue to you, as fairly and accurately as I can.

Those who are opposed to the use of stimulants, especially by children, often believe one or more of the following:

- Parents are giving their uncontrollable AD/HD children drugs to quiet them down, not for the child's sake but for their own peace of mind.
- Doctors and the pharmaceutical companies are in cahoots to boost sales of the drugs.
- There is little information about the safety or long-term use of stimulants.
- Stimulants are like cocaine and children are becoming high on the medications.
- Children can become addicted to the medications.
- Use of stimulants will make AD/HD children more likely to become drug addicts.

Safety was one of the main questions that I looked at when we were making our decision. Are these medications safe? Was I drugging my children? Would it make them high? When Theresa was first diagnosed, I didn't want to use stimulant medication to treat her AD/HD. I felt guilty as a parent that we were thinking of giving her a controlled substance. Then I began to read and study. What I discovered was the following scientific statistics on the use of stimulants. These statistics answered some of the questions for me about safety and the benefits of stimulants.

- Studies have shown that these medications, when used under medical supervision, are safe and extremely helpful to those with AD/HD.
- Seventy-five to 90 percent of children show moderate to significant improvement in AD/HD behaviors from the use of stimulants.
- Research indicates that when ingested in pill form in small to moderate doses, these medications do not create a high sensation but instead improve concentration.
- AD/HD children who are *not* treated for AD/HD with stimulants have *higher* drug abuse rates. Studies have shown that the prescribed use of these medications does not cause substance abuse problems— in fact, they seem to help prevent those with AD/HD from becoming drug addicts. Scientists haven't answered the "why" question yet. Perhaps it is because when receiving medication for their disorder, children are able to fit in a little better and behave more like normal children, thus avoiding some of the stressors, rejection, social isolation, and frustrations that AD/HD children experience.

Stimulants are not a cure for AD/HD. They help significantly, but they do not cure the disorder. Stimulants are a tool—a highly effective tool to help those with AD/HD cope with their disorder. Whether or not you choose to use stimulants to help treat your child's AD/HD is entirely up to you. Research the medications. Read both sides of the equation. Do the benefits outweigh the risks? This is a very difficult question and not all the answers are in yet. Be informed about your decision.

Does using these medications cause tics?

The use of stimulant medications by those with AD/HD can sometimes worsen tic disorders, such as Tourette's syndrome, and can uncover latent tic-like behaviors. Children who have a tic disorder as well as AD/HD are sometimes treated with Strattera or other nonstimulant medications.

Vocal tic disorders include behaviors such as throat clearing, snorting, sniffing, shouting, humming, and other odd vocalizations. Motor tics include eye blinking, facial grimaces, head jerking, and other odd physical movements. If your child experiences any of these symptoms after starting a stimulant medication, see your doctor.

Are generic versions of these medications available?

In some cases, yes. Whether or not a drug comes in a generic form can often make a difference in how much you (and your insurance company) will pay for the medication. Some insurance plans have a standard deductible, such as $5, $10, and $20 dollars. Other insurance plans will not cover brand-name drugs in the deductible price. For example, a generic drug might cost the buyer $10, while a brand-name drug would be $40.

Check with your pharmacy to see if a generic version is available. Keep in mind, however, that sometimes generic versions are not as effective as brand-name drugs.

Is medication necessary for treating AD/HD?

Is it helpful? Yes, very helpful. Is it necessary? Many experts believe that it is. Research has shown that stimulant medications help 75 to 90 percent of AD/HD children. Even the 75 percent statistic is an impressive percentage.

Can children take these medications?

Dextroamphetamine and amphetamine salts are recommended for children over the age of three. Methylphenidate and atomoxetine are recommended for children over the age of six.

Can preschool children take these medications?

According to a study in the *Journal of the American Medical Association,* 1 percent to 1.5 percent of two- to four-year-old children in the Medicaid system are receiving psychotropic drugs, including stimulants, antidepressants, or antipsychotic medications. An Intercontinental Medical Statistics study found a threefold increase in methylphenidate prescriptions in Canada and a tenfold increase in selective norepinephrine reuptake inhibitors in the United States in preschool children in recent years.

Although it is more commonplace for physicians to prescribe psychotropic medications to preschool children, please be careful about your decision on whether or not to give any of these medications for your young AD/HD child. Except for severe AD/HD, I personally do not think that these medications should be given to preschool children. All the facts are not in yet about the safety and benefits of stimulants on children this young.

Will my child's growth be stunted if he is treated with stimulants?

According to scientific studies, AD/HD children who are treated with stimulant medications experience slight weight and height differences, which some experts believe are unrelated to medication use.

Children who have been treated with stimulants for AD/HD experience a very small, 1- to 3-cm, difference in height. Other studies have shown that these height differences exist in younger children with AD/HD. In any case, by late adolescence, the same children catch up to their peers.

A recent study found that children who were treated with stimulants over a two-year period had average weights that were eight pounds lower than untreated children.

A common side effect of stimulant use is decreased appetite. According to the United States surgeon general, when an AD/HD child is treated with stimulant medications, regular monitoring of the child's height and weight is recommended.

How many children are receiving medication for AD/HD?

According to the 1995 National Disease and Therapeutic Index, physicians wrote 6 million prescriptions for stimulants and one million prescriptions for SNRIs for children in 1995. This estimates to 1.5 million schoolchildren, or 2.8 percent, who use stimulants to treat their AD/HD.

Other studies have shown a higher percentage. In a study in North Carolina, 9.5 percent of all school-aged children six to fourteen years of age received prescriptions for stimulants.

What are standard children's dosages for these medications?

How much medication your child receives daily depends on the personal results of medication use for your child. Perhaps there is significant improvement in your child's AD/HD symptoms with just a very small dose, or your child might need a larger dose to see the benefits of the medication. Dosage level does not always relate to age, weight, or symptom severity. Each child responds differently to medication. The National Institute of Mental Health is currently looking at ways to help refine the guidelines for "best dosage level," as well as helping parents and physicians find ways to manage the side effects of stimulant drug use. On pages 54–55 is a chart with standard dosage ranges for children ages six to fourteen.

How long will my child be on these medications?

For many years, it was thought that children somehow grow out of AD/HD. Now experts believe that AD/HD is a disorder that a person has his or her entire life.

Medication treatment is not a cure, it is a tool to help a person cope with his disorder. Some people learn how to use different parts of their brains to help them function. Other people have extensive organization tools to help them stay organized and focused. Also, when adults with AD/HD work in a field of interest to them, they stay on task and focused to a greater degree.

Continued treatment into adolescent and adulthood can be beneficial. Whether or not your child continues to use stimulants as an adult depends on how well they are functioning on their own, whether the medication has clear benefits, and of course, his or her own personal preference.

BRAND NAME	DAILY DOSAGE SCHEDULE	
Ritalin (short–acting)	2–3 times a day	
Methylin (short–acting)	2–3 times a day	
Ritalin SR (intermediate)	1 time a day	
Metadate ER	1 time a day	
Focalin	2 times a day	
Concerta (long–acting) **Metadate CD** (long–acting) **Ritalin LA** (long–acting) **Dexedrine** (short–acting)	1 time a day 1 time a day 1 time a day 1–2 times a day	
Adderall (intermediate)	1–2 times a day	
Dexedrine spansule	1–2 times a day	
Adderall–XR (long–acting)	1 time a day	
Strattera	1–2 times a day	

DURATION OF MED	DOSAGE AMOUNT
3-4 hours	5–20 mg each dose
3–4 hours	5–20 mg each dose
4–5 hours	20–40 mg in the morning or 40 mg a.m. and 20 mg p.m
4–5 hours	20–40 mg in the morning or 40 mg a.m. and 20 mg p.m.
4–5 hours	5–10 mg
10–12 hours	18–72 mg
7–8 hours	18–72 mg
8–12 hours	18–72 mg
4–5 hours	5–15 mg in the morning and 5–10 mg in the afternoon
4–5 hours	5–30 mg a.m. and/or 5–15 mg p.m.
5–8 hours	5–30 mg a.m. and/or 5–15 mg p.m.
10–12 hours	10–30 mg
5 hours	25–100 mg

How do we decide which medication is best for our AD/HD child?

Currently, there are no clinical characteristics to help predict which of the medications would be best for your child. Honestly, deciding which medication to use is a system of trial and error. Often, a patient will need to try different medications and dosages before a "winner" is found. As the child grows, the dosage will need to be changed. Often, too, a child will be started on a short-acting medication and graduate to a longer-lasting one.

Which medication you choose depends on the following:

- which medication seems to work the best
- any side effects experienced and the severity of the side effect
- ability to swallow pills
- any appetite-suppression problems experienced
- any embarrassment experienced by taking a pill at school
- any downtime problems experienced between doses
- sleeping difficulties
- the hours of coverage needed versus what the medication provides
- preference of the parent between a stimulant or an SNRI medication

If one medication doesn't work, don't give up. There is a 25 percent chance that another medication will work when the first choice doesn't. If "first-line" medications do not work to treat your child's AD/HD, there are also "second-line" medications to be considered, such as bupropion, nortriptyline, desipramine, clonidine, and guanfacine. It is best to try all first-line choices before considering other options. In addition, some patients find improvement with a combination of the various medications. Talk to your doctor about the various options available.

Should our AD/HD child take a "drug holiday" from medication use?

Some families choose to not give their child their AD/HD medication on the weekend or during the summer. The only value in doing this is to help you determine if the medication and dosage level are still working. AD/HD is a pervasive disorder. Untreated hours are potentially dangerous times for someone with AD/HD.

How do we know whether the medication is helping our AD/HD child?

Stimulant medications and atomoxetine often bring about improvements in the following areas:

- increased ability to pay attention
- increased ability to follow instructions
- fewer hyperactive behaviors
- fewer impulsive behaviors
- ability to sit at the dinner table, at school, at church, and other events
- ability to maintain eye contact during a conversation
- overall improved behavior
- improvements in school grades
- possible improvements in self-esteem
- possible improvements in social skills and peer relationships
- improvements in handwriting neatness and legibility

Are there some children who can't take these medications?

Yes. Some children experience side effects. These side effects can be either mild or severe and can include weight loss, tics, nausea, sleep problems, headaches, and (rarely) hallucinations. And approximately 10 to 30 percent of children with AD/HD do not respond to the first-line medications at all.

In these cases, there are other pharmaceutical options. Bupropion and imipramine—which are antidepressants—have been found to be helpful, although studies have shown that the medications are not as successful as stimulants. Clonidine is sometimes used for AD/HD children who have tic disorders and is sometimes used to aid sleep in AD/HD children. Neuroleptics, such as risperidone, can help improve AD/HD symptoms, but they can cause additional movement disorders.

Can use of these medications by children cause later drug abuse?

Studies have shown that AD/HD children who are treated with stimulants actually have lower rates of drug abuse problems than AD/HD children who are not treated with stimulants. It appears that the disorder itself is more responsible for future drug abuse problems than the treatment.

Children with AD/HD have an increased risk of abusing drugs and alcohol as adolescents and adults. However, a study conducted by the National Institute of Mental Health and the National Institute on Drug Abuse found that AD/HD boys who received stimulant treatment were much less likely to become alcohol and drug addicts. Later drug abuse problems are highly associated with the comorbid condition of conduct disorder (CD) rather than the treatment use of stimulant medications. Numerous other studies have also reached the same conclusion—that medication treatment for AD/HD decreases the risk for later drug and alcohol abuse.

Case reports of AD/HD children abusing their stimulant medications are rare. When abuses occur, it is often the child selling the drug or the parents' use and abuse of the child's prescription medication. Although case reports are rare, it does happen. This is why medications are usually locked away in a safe place in the school office.

Are stimulants controlled substances?

Yes. The prescriptions for stimulants must be picked up in person at the physician's office or mailed to your home on a monthly basis. When abused, these drugs can cause an increase in blood pressure and heart rate, feelings of exhilaration, and a high. Abuse of these medications can also lead to weight loss, heart failure, and death. Therefore, the distribution of these medications must be carefully "controlled."

5.

ALTERNATIVE
PRACTICES

. . . .

There are many, many alternative practices that can be helpful in treating AD/HD, but there are even more useless and harmful alternative practices. Be careful, in particular, of anyone who professes to be able to "cure" AD/HD.

What about special diets to treat AD/HD?

Wouldn't it be nice if there were some magical cure for AD/HD? Perhaps, if our child ate a certain type of food, or didn't eat another, his or her symptoms would disappear! Unfortunately, special diets have not been proven to be of any help in treating AD/HD.

There are many supposed dietary "cures" listed on the Internet. The Feingold diet is perhaps the most widely marketed dietary manipulation program. I, too, have considered special diets for our children and have done extensive research in this area. Below are a few issues of importance when considering the use of special diets to treat AD/HD:

- Over twenty different studies have been conducted to see if special diets can improve the symptoms of AD/HD.
- All of these studies determined that special diets have little or no effect on AD/HD symptoms.
- Controlled studies to date have demonstrated that sugar intake does not make children with AD/HD more hyperactive. (As a former teacher, I'm not so sure that I agree with this one!)
- Delaying treatment with medication while you try different diets robs your child of valuable time.
- Finally, if AD/HD is associated with smaller brain size in the prefrontal cortex, the basal ganglia, and the cerebellum, as current research has shown, diet will not change this. You cannot change the size and shape of someone's brain by changing what they eat.

Having said this, good nutrition is important for everyone. The American Heart Association has a set of guidelines to follow. And because stimulants can cause a decrease in appetite, nutrition should be closely monitored.

What about vitamins and minerals to treat AD/HD?

Vitamins and minerals are important to good health for both children and adults. When someone is treated with a stimulant, his or her appetite can also be affected, so a good multivitamin is essential for both AD/HD children and adults. Ask your physician or a nutritionist for a recommendation.

What about the use of medicinal herbs to treat AD/HD?

Although there are some natural herbs that can be helpful, such as Saint-John's-wort to treat depression, no herbs have been discovered yet to help the symptoms of AD/HD. Be careful of websites professing an herbal cure for AD/HD.

What about other complementary and alternative practices?

There are numerous complementary and alternative practices that can be used along with medication. For example, yoga is helpful in building strength, aiding in relaxation, and improving concentration and focus. Martial arts training can improve self-confidence and teach self-discipline. Massage can aid in relaxation and be used as a stress reducer. All of these alternative practices are helpful to the AD/HD child or adult.

Just as there are good alternative practices, there are even more expensive, useless, and even dangerous alternative therapies. Be careful of any alternative therapy that says it can cure your child's or your AD/HD. There are no cures for AD/HD. Not special diets, not energy field realignments, not heavy metal removal—none of these things will help control or cure the symptoms of AD/HD. AD/HD has a biological and genetic basis.

A few alternative practices that do not help in treating AD/HD include megavitamins, mineral supplements, EEG biofeedback (a proposed program to increase the amount of brain-wave activity), kinsesiology (this practice proposes to realign bones in the skull), treatment for infections (such as candida yeast), medications to treat inner ear problems (such as motion sickness medication), chelation therapy (a program that uses injections of crystalline acid to remove heavy metals from the system), or optometric vision training (proposes that defective eye movements cause AD/ HD behavioral problems). I repeat, none of these alternative practices are helpful, and some can be dangerous.

Before embarking on an alternative practice, be sure to consult your AD/HD physician.

6.

COPING WITH
THE DIAGNOSIS

. . . .

You just found out that your son has AD/HD. How do you help him cope? Should you tell anyone about his diagnosis? How about you? How do you cope? Coping with AD/HD isn't easy. A child might be embarrassed about his disorder. On the other hand, he might be relieved to finally know why he does what he does. You can help with this process.

HELPING YOUR CHILD COPE

Q Should I tell my child that he or she has AD/HD?

Yes, you should. Besides being aware of her disorder, she should play an active role in the treatment for her AD/HD.

Often children already know that something is wrong. As they mature, they begin to pick up on things. It might be the constant look of exasperation on a teacher's face, or low grades despite having studied, or cruel comments from peers. As a child gets older, she begins to internalize all the negative factors that can be a part of having AD/HD. If your child doesn't know that she has AD/HD, she begins to think thoughts such as "I'm stupid," "I can't get anything right," "Everyone hates me," or "I'm worthless." One of the largest problems with children with AD/HD is low self-esteem.

I can't stress enough how important it is that your child knows about his disorder and is involved in the treatment. I have known many people who were diagnosed as adults and felt a huge sense of relief. Finally, they know why they had problems in school. Finally, they understand why they keep "messing up" on the job. Finally, they understand why relationships are so difficult for them. At last, an answer to what's going on! And they found not only an answer but also direction on what steps to take. You can't fight something unless you know what you are fighting. It must have a face and a name. In this case, it's AD/HD. The tools to fight the disorder include medication, education about the disorder, love, patience, understanding, counseling, and coaching/adapting techniques.

Both of my girls know about their AD/HD. I explained the disorder to them in simple terms as soon as they were diagnosed. They know why they take their medications. They know why school is difficult for them. We talk about it and we work together to find solutions.

As they get older, they have been helpful in determining medication strengths, knowing when a medication needs to be increased or if it is too strong. We've also discussed and practiced techniques for making friends, following directions, and staying organized. When there is a problem, we talk about what happened and come up with a list of options that can be used in the future. By knowing about their AD/HD, they are aware of the difficulties and are a little more ready to meet them. We don't use the disorder as an excuse, however. When we talk about AD/HD, I tell them, "Everyone has something. If they don't, they will before their lives are over. Some people have more than one something. Some people have many somethings. Your something is AD/HD. It means you will have to work harder at paying attention than other people."

How can I help my child cope with AD/HD?

In 1998, the National Institute of Mental Health (NIMH) conducted a very large study on multimodal treatments of AD/HD. This study was called the Multimodal Treatment Study of AD/HD (or MTA). Researchers compared four different treatment options: stimulant medication alone, behavioral treatment alone, the combination of medication and behavioral treatments, and a control group (no treatment). After fourteen months, the combined treatment group showed significant improvements over both the behavioral treatment and the control group. Areas of improvement included social skill behaviors, parent/child relationships, anxiety levels, reading achievement, and aggressive/oppositional type behaviors. Parents also reported being more satisfied with the multimodal treatment approach, which also had some advantages for youths with AD/HD and co-morbid anxiety disorder.

Chapter 9 explains "The AD/HD Pyramid," a treatment strategy Dr. Van Haren and I created based on the recommendations of the National Institute of Mental Health.

Should I spend extra time with my AD/HD child?

Yes. Having AD/HD can be emotionally taxing for a child. They often experience failure at a higher rate than other children—both academically and socially. It is so important for you to be there for your child—physically, emotionally, and spiritually. Here are a few ways to bond with your AD/HD child:

- Go to as many of your child's music and sporting events as you possibly can manage.

- Cheer and clap loudly and profusely.
- Read to your child.
- Watch funny movies together.
- Toss a baseball, throw a Frisbee, or build a snowman together.
- Accompany your child on field trips.
- Have lunch with your child at her school. (If the school allows this, bring lunch for both of you!)
- Play games and laugh together.
- Talk, talk, and more talk.
- Go on a "Special Day with Mom or Dad."
- Accept your child for who he is. Don't expect your child to fit into your own expectations of what he should or shouldn't be—such as being an athlete, joining your fraternity, or attending your alma mater. Help him follow his dream, even if it isn't yours.

SPECIAL DAY WITH MOM OR DAD

· · · · · ·

A "Special Day with Mom or Dad" is a day when you spend some quality time with your child. This should include an activity of their choice, such as shopping, going to a movie, sledding, playing arcade games, or lunch at their favorite restaurant, and a small token of some sort, such as a toy, book, video game, or DVD. These tokens do not need to be expensive. For example, special days with Mom in the past have included a visit to Toys "R" Us, a day of window shopping, a movie, a trip to a museum, and enjoying a hamburger, fries, and a chocolate malt.

If your spouse or partner wants to be involved, have one "Special Day" in the fall for you and the child and another "Special Day" in the spring for your spouse or partner and the child. Don't run errands while you are on the special day. Dedicate the day to the importance and beauty of your lovely child. But if you have a special day during the school week, always arrange the day in advance with the school system. You'll want to avoid major test days or field trip days. Some days are more convenient for teachers than others.

Q Are there any children's books about AD/HD that you would recommend for my child?

Yes! Here are just a few to get you started:

- *Eagle Eyes: A Child's Guide to Paying Attention.* Jeanne M. Gehret. Fairport, NY: Verbal Images Press, 1996.
- *Eddie Enough!* Debbie Zimmitt. Rockville, MD: Woodbine House, 2001.
- *Eukee, the Jumpy Jumpy Elephant.* Cliff L. Corman and Esther Trevino. Plantation, FL: Specialty Press, 1995.
- *Jumpin' Johnny Get Back to Work! A Child's Guide to ADHD/Hyperactivity.* Michael Gordon. DeWitt, NY: GSI Publications, 1991.
- *Learning Disabilities and the Don't Give Up Kid.* (For both LD and AD/HD kids) J. Gehret. Fairport, NY: Verbal Images Press, 1990.
- *Learning to Slow Down and Pay Attention: A Book for Kids About ADD.* Kathleen G. Nadeau and Ellen B. Dixon. Annandale, VA: Magination Press, 1997.
- *Living with a Brother or Sister with Special Needs: A Book for Sibs.* D. Meyer, P. Vadasy, and R. Fewell. Seattle: University of Washington Press, 1985.
- *My Brother Matthew.* M. Thompson. Rockville, MD: Woodbine House, 1992.
- *Otto Learns About His Medicine: A Story About Medication for Children with ADHD.* Matthew R. Galvin. Washington, DC: American Psychological Association, 2001.
- *Putting On the Brakes: Activity Book for Young People with ADHD.* Patricia O. Quinn, Washington, DC: American Psychological Association, 1993.
- *Shelley, the Hyperactive Turtle.* Deborah M. Moss, Rockville, MD: Woodbine House, 1990.
- *Sparky's Excellent Misadventures: My A.D.D. Journal by Me (Sparky).*

Phyllis Carpenter. Washington, DC: American Psychological Association, 1999.

- *Zipper, the Kid with ADHD.* Caroline Janover. Rockville, MD: Woodbine House, 1997.

HELPING YOUR TEEN COPE

My teenager has just been diagnosed with AD/HD. How can I help him cope?

First of all, try to understand how your teenager is feeling. He might be angry with you or angry with himself. He might be embarrassed or depressed. He could be elated to finally know that there is a medical reason for what is going on and that he is not a bad, stupid, or lazy kid. If you have AD/HD, talk about your AD/HD with your teen. Tell him or her some of the difficulties you have had and how you have coped with them. If you have any humorous moments to relate, do that also.

Involve your teen in his treatment process. For more detailed information on helping your AD/HD teen, see Chapter 9.

Are there any books that you would recommend for my AD/HD teen?

Yes! Just a few include the following books for your teen and you (some are related to choosing a college):

- *Academic Success Strategies for Adolescents with Learning Disabilities and ADHD.* Esther H. Minskoff and David Allsopp. Baltimore: Paul H. Brookes, 2002.
- *ADD and the College Student: A Guide for High School and College Students with Attention-Deficit Disorder.* Patricia O. Quinn. Washington, DC: Magination Press/American Psychological Association, 2001.

- *The A.D.D. Hyperactivity Workbook for Parents, Teachers, and Kids.* H.C. Parker, D. Haynes, and J. Romanovich. Plantation, FL: Specialty Press, 1996.
- *Adolescents and ADD.* Patricia O. Quinn. Washington, DC: American Psychological Association, 1996.
- *Colleges with Programs for Students with Learning Disabilities or Attention Disorders.* Charles T. Mangrum and Stephen S. Strichart. Lawrence-ville, NJ: Peterson's, 2000.
- *Learning Outside the Lines: Two Ivy League Students with Learning Dis-abilities and ADHD Give You the Tools for Academic Success and Educa-tional Revolution.* Jonathan Mooney and David Cole. New York: Simon & Schuster, 2000.
- *Making ADHD a Gift.* Robert Evert Cimera. Boca Raton, FL: CRC Press, 2002.
- *Problem Solver Guide for Students with ADHD.* Harvey C. Parker. Plan-tation, FL: Specialty Press, 2001.
- *Survival Guide for College Students with ADD or LD.* Kathleen G. Nadeau. Washington, DC: American Psychological Association, 1994.

HELPING OTHER PEOPLE UNDERSTAND

My child's grandparents don't understand. They just think he is misbehaving. How do I help them understand AD/HD?

In defense of grandparents, they were raised in a generation where children were "seen but not heard." Children who didn't follow the rules were sometimes severely punished—for example, consider the old saying "Spare the rod, spoil the child." It is sometimes difficult for a person from that generation to understand an AD/HD child's behavior.

Just as having a child with AD/HD is a learning process for you, the same is true for other family members. All of us can learn and grow as the child learns and grows. It is important, however, that they understand the disorder, are supportive of your efforts, and are kind and patient with their grandchild. Start by having a positive, nonjudgmental talk with the child's grandparents. Tell them about the disorder. Tell them about what treatment options you have chosen. Tell them how they can help. Ask them if they have any suggestions. I would suggest encouraging them to read this book. Always listen to their suggestions with an open mind. Grandparents often have a wealth of knowledge and experience that you can draw upon to use with your AD/HD child.

Include them in your child's life. Invite them to your child's music performances and sporting events. Grandparents are great cheerleaders—even if their grandchild comes in tenth place.

Should I tell other people that my child has AD/HD?

With any medical condition, not everyone needs to know about it. The same is true with your child's AD/HD. If you do decide to tell another person, talk privately to the individual. Be honest, but also include some positive aspects on how your child is doing. The following people should be told about your child's disorder:

- Immediate family and extended family members. This group includes your significant other and the child's siblings, grandparents, aunts and uncles, and any other close family member. It is very important that this group be well informed and educated about AD/HD.
- School staff members. The child's primary teacher should be kept updated about the disorder and medication changes. Support teachers—such as music, art, and physical education teachers—should also be told. School secretaries are often the ones who give out the medications, so they should be told. If there is a problem, they are often the ones who call. Also, the school principal should be aware of your child's AD/HD.
- Day-care and after-school providers. If your work is outside of the home and your AD/HD child is in day care or before- and after-school care, this is another important group of people who should be

kept informed about your child's AD/HD. They spend a great deal of time with your child. They need to know why your child behaves the way he does and why he has problems with transitions. They should be willing to work with you to find positive solutions. They might even have a new idea or two!

- Close neighbors. Let's be frank here. Neighbors see a great deal of what goes on in your house or apartment. They hear a lot too! Neighbors can also be supportive and understanding about your child's disorder.

- Other significant people in your child's life. This group includes people such as camp counselors, Little League coaches, dance instructors, Girl Scout leaders, Sunday school teachers, and any other person who will be dealing with your child on a regular basis.

YOUR CHILD'S CHOICE

. . . . . .

As your child gets older, he or she may choose to tell close friends about his or her AD/HD. This is a personal decision. Don't do it for your child and don't push him or her in one direction or the other.

Let me tell you a story:

Our elementary school was going to have a carnival. Two of Theresa's friends were going to go around the carnival together without their parents. Theresa wanted to go with them. I agreed, as long as she checked in with me every 30 minutes. Her friends also had a stipulation: "That's great," they said. "But you'll need to keep your hyperactivity in check!" I was thrilled when I heard this. Number one, she had told them about her AD/HD. Number two, they were okay with it. Number three, they were able to talk about their concerns and limits in a positive way. Finally, Theresa asked me if she could take a "booster" pill (5 mg Ritalin) to help her manage her hyperactivity. The evening went very well. Theresa checked in with me, and she and her friends had a wonderful time.

HELPING YOURSELF COPE

Q Taking my AD/HD child to the grocery is a nightmare. She touches everything and asks for everything. How can I make this easier?

First of all, I suggest that you try to do your main grocery shopping without your AD/HD child. Grocery stores are an overload situation. There are tons of people pushing carts in every direction. There are music and lights and colorful signs. Everywhere you look there are advertisements and temptations for a child, right at eye level. You may try talking with them beforehand, having a reminder talk right before you go in the store, and offering a reward for good behavior. And still, they touch everything. They wander off. They ask for everything. It is just too difficult for an AD/HD child.

Try to do your main grocery shopping while the children are at school or in day care or while your partner watches them. When you do go to the grocery store with your AD/HD child, make sure he has had his medication, and get only ten items or fewer. The quicker you are, the fewer temptations and distractions your child will have. Offer a reward of some sort for not touching and not asking for items. This could include a bagel, a doughnut, a ride on the mechanical horse, a comic book, or a small trinket from a vending machine. Be careful of giving candy or too many sweets, because they aren't good for their bodies or their teeth. Don't expect perfection. Practice makes perfect. As they get older, they will get better at this and you will be able to take them on longer excursions.

Q I'm losing my mind with my AD/HD child
or teenager. How do I personally cope
with this disorder?

I remember when I was pregnant with my first child, one of my friends
who already had children said, "Oh boy, this will change your life!" I
thought, *Oh, maybe just a little.* Now just going to the grocery to get a jug
of milk is a major outing!

Having an AD/HD child can amplify the stressors of parenthood. According to research, parents of AD/HD children express a greater level of
unhappiness as a parent than parents of non-AD/HD children.

So what can you do? Here are a couple of suggestions that might help
you keep your sanity:

- First of all, try to stay calm and patient. I pray for patience every
  morning when I am taking my shower.
- Try to keep things in perspective. If your child won't do his home-
  work today, it's not the end of the world. (Besides, he needs to learn
  that there are consequences for not turning in assignments.)
- Use humor as much as possible.
- Take frequent breaks. This can include a brisk walk, a hot bath, or a
  night out with friends. Even a short minute or two outside on the
  porch can help perk you up—especially in cold weather.
- When, and not if, you become discouraged, talk with a good friend.
  Just be sure not to do it in front of your child.
- Do something fun and silly by yourself, with your spouse, or with
  your children. Build a snowman, climb a tree, take a walk in the rain
  and splash in the puddles.
- Prepare a mental "gratitude list" during the day.
- Drop your housekeeping standards a bit.
- Stop caring so much about what people think. Do the best you can
  and go on.
- Before you get home or pick up your children, stop for a minute or
  two and collect your thoughts.

THE GRATITUDE LIST

. . . . . .

A few years ago, when I was still teaching, I found myself constantly complaining and being negative about everything. One afternoon, as I was driving home from work, I found myself complaining nonstop. *Why did I have to work at a place across town? Why couldn't I stay home? Why did it have to snow today? Why couldn't I have a better car? Why did this guy in front of me have to go so slow?* This list went on and on. Suddenly, an elderly woman stepped out from a sidewalk and traffic came to a standstill as she slowly crossed the road. I was in such a bad mood that I thought, *Why does she have to be out on a day like today?* I stopped and realized what I was thinking, what an awful rut I had gotten into, and what a terrible person I was becoming as a result. I decided then and there to prepare a mental gratitude list during the day—things or people or experiences from that day for which I was grateful. Very quickly, my attitude began to change. I would wake up and it would be raining. *Oh, doesn't the rain smell nice,* I would think, and I would add that to my mental gratitude list. Soon I was noticing things that I hadn't before—a cute dog barking out a car window, the nice cashier who smiled at me, the warm socks I was wearing in my boots, and the solitary daffodil sticking its head up through the snow. Every day, as I drove home from work, I would go over the gratitude list in my head for that day.

When you have a child with AD/HD, it is essential that you keep a positive attitude. Techniques such as this will help you to stay sane.

Our child's AD/HD is creating problems in our marriage. What should we do?

Marriage can be very difficult, as we know by the high rate of divorce in this country. Any crisis—such as losing a job, chronic illness in the family, or having a child with disabilities—can push a marriage over the edge. It's not just the AD/HD; it's life in general. Sometimes we have more than we can handle.

For your sake and the sake of your children, it is important to try to work out any difficulties you might have. Here is a list to help you get started:

- Go on frequent dates. Get to know each other again. Don't talk about the children, work difficulties, financial strains, or relationship problems when you go out.
- Do something romantic and unexpected. Have a picnic on a snowy day. Climb a tree together. Rent a canoe and spend the afternoon just being quiet. It's amazing sometimes how little it can take to rejuvenate a relationship.
- Take turns talking. When your spouse talks, listen.
- If your spouse takes care of most of the housework and child-rearing responsibilities, give her or him the night off.
- Leave kind, appreciative notes around the house and in the car.
- Each week, have a family meeting to discuss any problems or important family events and to give kudos for a "job well done."
- Get plenty of rest. Fatigue always makes things worse.
- Try to maintain a "unified front" when dealing with discipline or behavior problems with your child.
- Don't blame each other for the problems with your AD/HD child.
- Don't blame your AD/HD child or your other children for problems in your marriage.
- Tell your spouse or significant other, "You're doing a great job." Or "You're a great parent."
- Be willing to say, "What can I do to help?"
- If your spouse thinks you have AD/HD, get tested. There is a very strong genetic link with AD/HD. He or she might be right.
- If you have AD/HD, be appreciative of your spouse. Keep in mind how hard it might be for him or her to deal with the difficulties of the disorder.
- If your spouse has AD/HD, be patient and understanding. Love him or her unconditionally.
- There is nothing wrong with seeing a marriage or family counselor. Knowing when you need counseling and being willing to ask for help are signs of courage and strength.

What organizations are available to help with our child's AD/HD?

The largest national nonprofit organization to help AD/HD children, parents, teachers and schools, professionals, and AD/HD adults is Children and Adults with Attention-Deficit/Hyperactivity Disorder (CHADD). CHADD provides members with the following:

- General facts on AD/HD.
- Information on who qualifies for special education services under the Individuals with Disabilities Education Act and Section 504 of the Rehabilitation Act.
- Referrals to local CHADD chapters, which hold seminars with expert speakers, work with local teachers and school systems, and sponsor support groups of both parents of AD/HD children and adults with AD/HD.
- A subscription to *Attention!*, a bimonthly publication that offers helpful suggestions on dealing with AD/HD and reports on the latest research about the disorder. The magazine is worth every penny of the $45 yearly family fee for CHADD membership.
- CHADD also sponsors the CHADD National Resource Center. The center is an information and referral service.

I highly recommend CHADD as one of the first steps in your journey with AD/HD. The organization's motto is "CHADD cares"—and it shows! (Contact information for CHADD can be found in the website resource section on page 180.)

Some other organizations that provide support include:

- ADDvance (a resource for women and girls with attention-deficit disorders): www.addvance.com
- Attention Deficit Disorder Association (ADDA): (484) 945-2101 or www.add.org

- Attention Deficit Information Network (Ad-IN): (781) 455-9895 or
  www.addinfonetwork.com
- NAMI (formerly called National Alliance for the Mentally Ill):
  (800) 950-NAMI or www.nami.org
- Parent Advocacy Coalition for Educational Rights (PACER):
  (952) 838-9000 or www.pacer.org

I also strongly encourage you to sign up for "Attention Research Update." This is a free e-mail newsletter that is highly informative and helps
keep you updated on the latest research and findings. You can sign up for
this service at www.helpforadd.com.

7.

EDUCATIONAL ISSUES

. . . .

Sometimes, one of the first people to "unofficially" diagnose a child with AD/HD is the classroom teacher. He usually has a great deal of experience with children. He is trained in the education of children and can quickly spot differences in learning styles and behavior. Having taught numerous students allows the teacher to observe that your child's behaviors are similar or dissimilar to other behaviors that he has seen previously. When your child's behavior mimics previous AD/HD children's behaviors, "red lights" flash in the teacher's mind. The teacher can often pinpoint the disorder before the parents can, because he has experienced it many times previously with other students. AD/HD is a common disorder. Usually one or two students per class have it!

Your AD/HD child has legal rights concerning his AD/HD and his education. And besides home, school is where he spends most of his time. His experiences there can make him or break him. As a parent, you can help your child receive the very best education possible.

What are my child's legal rights?

There are two federal laws that guarantee a "free, appropriate education" (FAPE) for children with disabilities.

The first law is Section 504 of the Rehabilitation Act of 1973. Section 504 is a *civil rights law.* Because schools receive federal funds, it prohibits them from "discriminating against children with disabilities" and requires that these organizations "provide disabled children with reasonable accommodations." The key word under this law is "reasonable." If a child's ability to learn is substantially limited because of AD/HD, they will qualify under Section 504—even if they are not in a special education classroom.

A child is not automatically qualified under Section 504. The school must decide that the child's disability substantially limits his or her ability to perform in the classroom.

Under Section 504, the school must:

- Give "written assurance" that a child is not being discriminated against.
- Choose an employee to "coordinate compliance."
- Provide "notice of nondiscrimination" in their student and parent handbooks.
- Provide parents with "procedural safeguards." These include chances to review the child's records and the right to have an impartial hearing about their child's disability, placement, and testing procedures.

Section 504 does not:

- Require parents to give permission for testing, although parents must be notified verbally that testing will take place.
- State how often the testing should occur.
- Demand that outside evaluations from physicians and psychiatrists play a role in the school's evaluation process.

Before a child is qualified under Section 504, he or she must have received an evaluation from the school. Children with milder forms of AD/HD are usually covered under Section 504.

The second federal law is the Individuals with Disabilities Education Act (IDEA). IDEA is an *education law.* Evaluations under IDEA are much more complex and involve a multidisciplinary approach. To receive special education services under IDEA, your child must have "ADHD that results in a heightened alertness to stimuli in the classroom that limits alertness to academic tasks." Your child's AD/HD must be "long-lasting (chronic) or have a substantial impact (acute)." The key words here are *heightened alertness, chronic,* and *acute.*

Under IDEA, schools must:

• Provide a free, appropriate education to all children with disabilities.
• Conduct an in-depth evaluation of children with AD/HD. This includes reviewing grades, reports on behavioral problems, and any assessment tests that have been conducted.
• This evaluation must include at least one teacher and one other outside specialist—for example, your pediatrician.
• Conduct the evaluation without undue delay.
• Have the parents' permission before conducting any evaluations.
• Consider any other reports or evaluations that the child has received from other agencies, schools, or physicians.
• Identify all of the child's needs.
• Conduct a reevaluation of the child's needs every three years.
• Allow parents to request a hearing to challenge the school's decisions. For example, if the school determines that your child doesn't need special help in reading and you disagree, you are guaranteed a meeting to challenge their decision. They must notify you of the meeting in writing.

Children with more severe forms of AD/HD often qualify under IDEA. Usually a child's attention-deficit/hyperactivity disorder will qualify under one of these two federal laws.

You can find out more about Section 504 and IDEA at the following websites:

- Children and Adults with Attention–Deficit/Hyperactivity Disorders (www.chadd.org/facts/add_facts04.htm; www.chadd.org/legislative/ idea_final_regs.htm; and www.chadd.org/legislative/ideaq-a.htm)
- "A Guide to Section 504: How it applies to students with Learning Disabilities." Learning Disabilities Association of America (www .ldanatl.org)
- "Overview of ADA, IDEA, and Section 504." ERIC Digest E537, Educational Resources Informational Center (www.ed.gov/databases/ ERIC_Digests/ed389142.html)

What is an IEP?

Under IDEA, AD/HD children are eligible to receive an individualized education plan (IEP). This plan:

- Requires that a child continue to be educated in a standard class that follows the regular academic curriculum. This is a requirement about the instructional program, not the location of the classroom.
- Requires the school to define your child's "current level of performance" and how the AD/HD "affects progress" of your child's education.
- Requires "measurable annual goals" to ensure that your child is progressing.
- Requires a list of any "modifications required" for your child, such as a teacher reading the questions from a test to your child rather than your child taking the test on his own.
- Requires a list of classroom activities in which your child will not participate (for example, not participating in the regular classroom reading project and instead being pulled out into a special reading group).
- Requires the school to keep records of all important information, such as the date services began, dates and length of meetings, who attended the meetings, the location of special services, and any changes that are made to the plan.

- Requires the school to prepare a description of how it will measure your child's progress and how you will be notified of this progress.
- Requires the school to prepare "transition services" when your child reaches the age of fourteen. This is to help your special education child prepare for work and additional education.
- Requires that the school review the IEP once a year.

Does my AD/HD child have to be placed in a special classroom?

No. IDEA has a special clause called least restrictive environment, or LRE. This means that if your child can function in a regular classroom (with a few adaptions), he or she should be put in a regular classroom.

How can I help my child's teacher understand his AD/HD?

I know how difficult it is to be a teacher. Teachers are underpaid and not appreciated as much as they should be. They put in endless hours of preparation work and attend hundreds of meetings. Art, music, foreign language, computer training, and physical education teachers see the entire school population during the year. This can add up to hundreds of children (or thousands at the upper levels). These teachers are expected to know all of the children's names and how they are progressing—not to mention medical problems, learning disabilities, asthma, allergies to certain foods, problems at home, and so on. You can see what a monumental task this is! So I understand, to a certain extent, how having a child with special needs can push a teacher beyond what he or she is capable of handling.

Here are a few guidelines to help you and your child's teacher (or teachers) work cooperatively for the benefit of your AD/HD child:

- Many schools allow parents to request certain characteristics in their child's upcoming teacher. If possible, meet with all the classroom teachers for that upcoming year and find out a little about their educational philosophies and personalities. Questions that you might ask include: "How long have you been teaching?" "What is your philosophy of education?" "How do you deal with behavior problems in the classroom?" "What methods have you used in the past to help AD/HD children?"
- If your child receives a teacher that views your child as a problem, request a different teacher.
- Go to all parent/teacher meetings.
- During conferences, meet with the secondary teachers as well (art, music, etc.).
- Volunteer whenever you can to help with classroom projects.
- Volunteer to go on as many field trips as possible.
- Help with classroom parties.
- Keep in regular contact with your child's teacher about his or her progress.
- Be supportive when any problems occur.
- Offer suggestions about behavioral plans or techniques that work at home.
- Listen, with an open mind, about any ideas your child's teacher has.
- Be flexible.
- Help the physical education teacher with field day. Help the art teacher with art projects. Help the music teacher with music programs. I realize that many parents work and can't help very often. Volunteering one or two days a year can make a difference.
- Praise the teacher for her efforts. Let her know how much you appreciate her hard work. Small gifts or tokens of appreciation are always nice. A gift certificate to her favorite restaurant or store is also helpful. Some schools have strict rules about a "public servant," including teachers, accepting gifts. It's best to check with your child's school system on their particular guidelines and rules before purchasing anything.
- Acknowledge that teaching an AD/HD child is difficult.
- If you have a criticism, try to present it in a nonjudgmental way.

According to a 2004 survey of 1,018 Michigan teachers by the Michigan Education Association, the number-one item teachers wanted was more contact with parents. Sixty-five percent of teachers reported that they encouraged parent visits to the classroom, and 82 percent said they would welcome suggestions from parents. So talk to your child's teacher. Make appointments to visit the classroom. Offer to help the teacher with school projects. Finally, write notes, phone, or use e-mail on a weekly basis with your child's teacher.

What should I do if my child's teacher is not supportive?

If your child's classroom teacher is not supportive, request a new teacher. But first try to work with all the teachers your child sees in a kind, supportive manner. If there is a problem with their understanding of your child's disorder, offer suggestions. If you feel the teacher is being harsh and unsupportive of your child, you might need to discuss the situation with the school principal. There are many wonderful teachers out there who are supportive, understanding, and kind. There are others who think of teaching as just a paycheck and your child as a problem. These teachers can permanently damage your child's self-esteem. It is very important that you don't allow that to happen. Helping your child maintain a positive attitude about school and education is essential.

HOW SCHOOLS CAN HELP

· · · · · ·

Let me give you a couple of short personal examples of how our school team works together to benefit our children. All of our children's primary teachers have been very supportive and help us monitor medication side effects and dosage amounts. Last year, my younger daughter Jenny's first-grade teacher called to ask if she had taken her medication that morning. "Yes," I replied, "I handed her the pill this morning." "Well, I just wondered because she is really having a difficult time paying attention and is extremely off-task today," she told me.

I hung up the phone and thought about it a little bit. Then I walked over to where Jenny ate breakfast and looked under the table. There on the floor was her pill. This was not the only day she didn't take her medication, and her teacher always knew.

On another day, I waited and waited for one of my girls to come home from the bus stop. She never showed. I called the school secretary, who immediately called the bus driver. Within three minutes the school called to say she'd gotten off the bus as usual. I took a tour through the neighborhood and found her taking the long, "scenic" route home.

The point of both these stories is that because I knew the school staff well, we were able to immediately pinpoint the problem, whether it was medication or easing my worries.

8.

LIFESTYLE ISSUES

. . . .

Problems with homework seem like almost a daily issue with our family. Often, the kids don't want to do it, have a hard time focusing, or forgot their worksheets and books. The day-to-day issues that your family faces can be the most difficult and the most frustrating—problems with homework, fighting with siblings, making friends, and of course, the special issues you face with your AD/HD teen! This chapter will offer suggestions to make your life a little easier.

HOMEWORK

Doing homework with my child is a nightmare. How can we make this easier?

Boy, do I understand this! Here are a couple of helpful suggestions:

• Give your AD/HD child a 30-minute break when she is first home from school. When you get home from work, you're tired. You want to sit down, read the paper, watch television, have a snack, or walk the dog. The last thing you want to do is to immediately start working again, so don't expect that from your child.

- Have a small healthy snack and a drink available.
- Keep a regular homework time every night (for example, beginning at 5 p.m.). Set an alarm. When the alarm rings at 5, it's time to start homework. It might take your child a little while to get used to this schedule, and she might complain and whine at first.
- For younger children, supervise them and help them with their homework. For teens, work in the same area that they are in (for example, the kitchen table) so you are available if they need you. You can also see that they are staying on task.
- When your child is finished, review the homework for accuracy and neatness.
- Have your child make any changes that are necessary and have her place the homework back in the appropriate place in her backpack.
- When your child is finished, he is free to do a fun activity.
- If the homework has not been completed in a reasonable amount of time, wake him up early in the morning to finish. AD/HD children often take longer than average children to complete an assignment. If you force them to work for a long period of time to finish, they will become angry and the situation could get worse. Use the early morning time as "special time"—a time with just the two of you to talk, eat breakfast, and finish homework.
- If possible, work with only one child at a time on homework.
- Schools have a general rule regarding how much homework a child should receive each night—about 15 minutes for each grade level. So first-graders receive 15 minutes, second-graders receive 30 minutes, and so on. If your second-grader is receiving an hour of homework each night, you might want to talk with the teacher.
- Keep in touch with the teacher about tests and large assignments. AD/HD children often need more time to prepare for a test or to complete a project or report. If you know about these assignments in advance, that helps.
- Break large assignments up into smaller units. For example, to pre-

pare for a test, read the chapter on one day, outline the chapter on a second day, study the outline on a third and fourth day.

- Start early on large assignments with your child. Don't wait until the last minute.
- To memorize important facts, I take a copy of the information along in the car. On occasions, at the store or while we are driving, I will ask my daughter to remember one or two facts. For example, I might have her recite a spelling word while we are driving to the store. When we arrive, I might have her spell it again or a different spelling word. Homework facts can be reinforced throughout the week in small ways.
- Homework should be part of your child's incentive chart for the week. (Sample Incentive Charts can be found in Appendix A.)

My child is constantly forgetting to bring his homework home. What should I do?

Don't get angry. This is to be expected as a part of his or her disorder. That doesn't make it acceptable, but it is very understandable. Your goal is to help him learn ways to successfully cope with his disorder. For school, coping tools include planners, charts, and extra books. Here are a few things to help you with this task:

- If your school has extra books available, ask to borrow or purchase subject books for home use.
- Purchase a school organizer for your child. This could include a binder that has a small calendar, a pocket folder, and an assignment notebook. Another great idea is to purchase an accordion-style folder with eight to ten insert areas. Each insert area can be labeled with a different subject. Therefore, the child has all his materials with him when he comes home! (Thank you, Melissa Smith, for this wonderful suggestion!)
- The assignment notebook should be signed by his teacher (or by him if he is older) each afternoon before leaving school. The assign-

ment notebook should have a box on each page for "materials needed."

- Make friends with the custodian so you can get into the school if necessary.
- If your child forgets materials, this should be reflected on his incentive chart (see Appendix A).
- If your child says he doesn't have any homework, don't assume he is right. AD/HD children often forget. Make sure and check.
- Don't get angry with your child. If your child is taught organizational skills, he will learn how to use them. He will also, you hope, mature, and this will become less of a problem area. Remember to be positive and helpful.

STAYING UPRIGHT IN THE MIDST OF THE STORM

. . . . . .

Pray or meditate for strength and patience every day.
Offer lots of encouragement to your child.
Practice forgiveness and tolerance.
Remember the word *flexibility*.
Give your child lots of love! And more love!

SAFETY

My child is too rough with his siblings, friends, and pets. What can we do?

There are numerous reasons your AD/HD child might be too rough. These include the following:

- the impulsive/hyperactive aspect of the disorder
- proprioceptive sensory difficulties
- other comorbid disorders, such as conduct disorder

There are certain things that you can do to help your child learn to be gentle with peers and animals. First of all, medication is helpful. The medications for AD/HD help improve impulsive/hyperactive behaviors. If your AD/HD child also has conduct disorder, there are additional medications to help in that area. The Wilbarger Protocol for Deep Touch Pressure can also help improve proprioceptive difficulties.

Besides helping your child learn appropriate behaviors, it is also important that you protect his siblings, his friends, and any animals or pets with which your child has contact. It isn't fair to brothers and sisters to be constantly hit, pushed, shoved, and teased. You owe it to them to provide them with a safe and happy home life. Try to follow these guidelines:

- Do not leave your aggressive AD/HD child unsupervised at any time.
- Whenever possible, remain within the same vicinity as your child. For example, if your children are playing in the backyard, do some gardening work there.
- If your child hurts someone, put the child in time-out. After the time-out period is finished, talk with your child about how that behavior hurt someone. Discuss options and then briefly practice an appropriate behavior. Your child should also apologize to the offended party, and make restitution. It is very easy to say that you are sorry. Making restitution or doing something to make amends is essential!
- Reinforce the idea to your child that having a pet is a privilege. Before buying a pet, do research with your child about the animal. Learn its traits, habits, and behaviors. Learn how to take care of the pet. After the pet has been purchased, supervise its care closely. Do not just assume that your AD/HD child is giving it food and water. You might have to supervise its care daily in ways such as watching your child feed or water the pet. Do not allow your child to mistreat the animal. If he does, remove the pet from the home. You might be able to try again when your AD/HD child is a little older. You might want to think about allowing your AD/HD child to have contact with a larger, "sturdier" animal. Horseback riding lessons are an excellent way to teach appropriate behaviors with animals. It also helps somewhat with tactile defensive issues. It's also a lot of fun!

What safety issues should we be aware of with our AD/HD child?

AD/HD children are at a much greater risk of injury than children without AD/HD. They have more accidents on a bicycle, while skating, and even while walking. AD/HD children have much higher medical costs than non-AD/HD children and have more trips to the hospital's emergency room. A lack of attention might cause an AD/HD child not to see a car coming. An impulsive behavior could include suddenly doing a back flip into a shallow end of the pool. Excessive hyperactivity could cause an AD/HD child to go faster than he can physically control himself.

So what can you do? Here are a few helpful suggestions:

- Always try to remain in the same room or vicinity as your AD/HD child.
- If the child is taking a bath, sit on the toilet seat and catch up on some reading.
- Make sure your child wears the proper safety equipment (helmets, kneepads, etc.) when he is using a bike, skateboard, or skates.
- Before you put the car in drive, check to see that your AD/HD child is in the car and buckled up.
- Keep an emergency first aid kit in your home.
- Keep harmful tools (such as knives, saws, and power tools), chemicals, and firearms out of the reach of children.
- Review pedestrian safety rules often with your AD/HD child.

Coaching lessons about safety are found in Chapter 10.

SOCIAL

Q My child has trouble making and keeping friends. How can we help her socially?

This is a major area of difficulty for the AD/HD child and teen. Problems in this area often stretch into adulthood. Below are some suggestions:

- Listen to your child and the problems that she is having. Discuss them with her.
- Never blame her. Never say things like "If your behavior wasn't so lousy, maybe you would have some friends" or "No wonder no one likes you!" AD/HD is difficult enough; she doesn't need guilt and sadness added on top of it.
- Let her know that you are a team. If she tells you there is a problem, say, "Okay, we'll figure this out together."
- Don't always assume it is something that he is or isn't doing. It might have nothing to do with his actions.
- Allow your child to have frequent encounters with other children. If you live in a secluded area, arrange numerous play dates.
- Throw a party! It doesn't have to be a birthday party. Arrange a "Godzilla Party," complete with a Godzilla cake, monster face painting, and a viewing of one of the old (and cheesy) Godzilla movies.
- If your young child is having problems with a particular child, invite the child and parent over for a play date.
- If your child is being teased or harassed by another child, talk to the teacher or the parent. Don't allow your child to be bullied.
- Involve your child in different activities where there are different children. For example, church or synagogue children's groups, dance lessons, soccer teams, Girl and Boy Scouts, and environmental clubs. If your child is being rejected by peers at school, having friends from a different group can help.
- If your child still has problems, you should involve the expertise of a

psychologist, social worker, or counselor. This individual can assist your child to help identify any problem areas, as well as teaching social skill techniques and problem-solving skills.

- If your child is depressed about social problems, he might need an antidepressant. You can talk to your AD/HD specialist about any problems your child is experiencing in this area.

Coaching lessons for social skills are found in Chapter 10.

Do AD/HD teenagers have a higher risk of developing substance problems?

Studies have shown that AD/HD teens who do not receive medication for this disorder are at a substantially higher risk for substance abuse than non-AD/HD teens. Studies have also shown that when AD/HD teens receive medication treatement, the risk level goes down to the abuse rate for their non-AD/HD peers. When a medicated AD/HD teen is involved with drugs, it is usually by selling his or her medication rather than using illegal drugs.

Another issue involved is conduct disorder. When an AD/HD teen has conduct disorder as well, their risk for drug abuse increases.

Should someone with AD/HD drink alcoholic beverages?

A 1998 study conducted by Dr. Timothy Wilens of Harvard Medical School found that substance abuse disorders appear at an earlier age in those with AD/HD and are much more severe. The study also found that AD/HD adults with substance abuse problems who go through an alcohol treatment program are less likely to recover.

Experts believe that the difficulties adults have had with academic underachievement, social awkwardness, and feelings of failure and demoralization can lead to substance abuse. Other experts believe that drug users with AD/HD are looking for ways to self-medicate so they can improve their concentration levels and experience relief from feelings of inadequacy, sadness, and depression. AD/HD individuals who abuse alcohol are looking for ways to unwind and relax.

Because of the high abuse risks, it is very important that your AD/HD teen does not drink or use drugs.

For many years, I was a casual, "social" drinker. I would have a drink or two on special occasions. When I discovered the high rate of substance abuse for AD/HD teens, I realized that I would be asking my children never to drink. At that point, I made a major commitment. I decided that I couldn't ask them to do something that I wasn't doing. So I quit drinking. This may be a commitment you'll want to make.

Are there any issues with driving a car with which we should be concerned?

Yes. According to the National Highway Traffic Safety Administration, highway crashes are the number-one cause of death of young people ages fifteen to twenty. Studies have shown that teens with AD/HD have even more automobile accidents and traffic citations than teens without AD/HD. In addition, AD/HD teens have a higher risk of being involved in a serious traffic accident.

Below is a list of items to keep in mind with your AD/HD teen and driving privileges:

- Driving is a privilege. Please stress this with your teen.
- AD/HD teens should go through an extensive driver's training course.
- Have your teen fill out a driving contract. (One is provided for you in Appendix B.)
- Make sure that you have substantial insurance coverage in the event of an accident. Additional "umbrella" liability policies help protect your family from personal injury lawsuits.
- AD/HD teens should take stimulant or atomoxetine medications to treat their AD/HD.
- Longer-lasting medications, or adding a second dose of medication,

should be seriously considered for your AD/HD teen to cover the evening hours.

- Stress the importance with your teen of not drinking when driving or planning to drive.

- Your AD/HD teen should drive a safe car. I would recommend a larger automobile with "bend" room. Smaller, compact cars don't do well in accidents. I would also recommend one with both driver- and passenger-side air bags. Be careful also of SUVs, which have a high rollover rate.

- Set a rule where only one or two other passengers can ride in the vehicle with your AD/HD teen. You've heard the phrase "The more, the merrier." Well, with teens, and not just AD/HD teens, the more teens there are in the vehicle, the riskier it is. AD/HD teens in particular might be distracted by all the noise and talk. They might also impulsively do something foolish to show off.

- Try not to overreact if your AD/HD teen has an accident. Cars can be replaced. Your child can't be. However, part of the child's contract with you should state that he or she is responsible for any repairs, after insurance, to the car.

Should our AD/HD teen be allowed to babysit?

Because of the inattention, impulsivity, and hyperactivity, as well as other comorbid disorders, most AD/HD children are not ready for babysitting jobs at the standard ages that other children are. It depends on the child, but I would suggest waiting until your AD/HD child is fifteen or sixteen rather than thirteen or fourteen before considering allowing her or him to babysit. Babysitting is a huge responsibility and should not be taken lightly. Babysitters must pay close attention to their charges and be able to think through situations quickly. You might consider signing your child up for a babysitting course at a local hospital to learn infant CPR.

9.

PULLING IT ALL TOGETHER:
THE AD/HD PYRAMID

. . . .

AD/HD is a difficult disorder to handle. There is not one stand-alone solution. Some people think that if they change their child's diet, the AD/HD will be cured. Others believe that medication alone is the answer. Medication helps a great deal, but it is only part of the equation.

In 1998, the National Institute of Mental Health (NIMH) released results of a very important study on AD/HD. The NIMH Multimodal Treatment Study of ADHD, also called the MTA Study, followed 576 AD/HD children for fourteen months and compared the results of various treatment methods. The study compared AD/HD children who were receiving medication alone, behavioral treatment alone, and both medication and behavior treatment and a control group that was not receiving treatment. The MTA Study found that the combined treatment method was significantly superior to the behavioral treatment alone and the control group. Using medication only to treat AD/HD also had a high score, although not as high as the multimodal treatment. Significant improvements with this combined treatment were recorded in parent/teacher relationships, anxiety, reading achievement levels, social skills, oppositional and aggressive behaviors, and parent satisfaction levels with the results of treatment.

A multimodal treatment plan is definitely the best way to go! But what treatments should be included in the management of my child's AD/HD? What exactly is a "multimodal" program?

Dr. Van Haren and I have worked a great deal to define what constitutes an effective AD/HD multimodal program. We combined his background in child psychiatry and AD/HD, my experiences as a teacher, the coaching lessons my mother used when teaching my autistic brother, and the results from the NIMH study. In this next section, Dr. Van Haren and I have "pulled it all together" for you with "The AD/HD Pyramid."

The first layer of the pyramid includes the AD/HD specialist/team leader, the parents, the teacher, and the AD/HD child. These areas are very important. You can't build the rest of the pyramid without them.

The second layer can also be very helpful. It includes counseling (individual, family, or marriage), academic modifications, and occupational and alternative therapies.

The third layer includes just two very important items: coaching and behavioral modification charts. (The actual coaching lessons can be found in Chapter 10; behavior modification charts are in Appendix A.)

Last but not least is the top layer of the pyramid—medication. Medication is extremely helpful and an essential part of the AD/HD pyramid.

I have listed these items throughout the book, but here they are brought together in one useful diagram. Each block is important. If you remove one block from a pyramid, it begins to wobble. Remove two and the structure collapses.

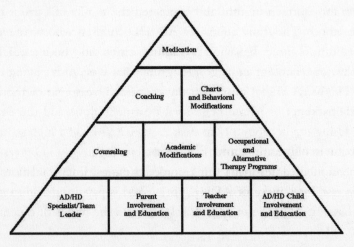

FIRST LAYER

There is an African story called "It Takes a Village" (to raise a child). How right this story is! And with an AD/HD child, even more so. AD/HD can be a very difficult disorder to handle. It takes everyone working together in a positive, constructive way for treatment to be successful. The list could include the AD/HD specialist, the parents and stepparents, therapists, coaches, teachers, day-care providers, grandparents, aunts, uncles, neighbors, siblings, and the AD/HD child. The more positive, encouraging people your child has on his team, the greater his chances for success. With everyone's help, he can grow up to be a happy, well-adjusted, productive member of society.

AD/HD Specialist/Team Leader

Your AD/HD specialist should serve as the team leader. He or she should diagnose the disorder and any comorbid disorders, prescribe and monitor medication use, and help determine suggested treatment options, including occupational therapy or family counseling. If you don't already have an AD/HD specialist, ask your pediatrician for a couple of referrals. You can talk to other parents with AD/HD children to find out which specialist they use and who they would recommend. Find someone who is highly qualified and knowledgeable about the disorder. Also, both you and your child should feel comfortable with the person. After all, this is going to be a very long relationship. A few questions to ask when you are interviewing the AD/HD specialist: What university did you attend? How long have you been practicing? What percentage of your patients have AD/HD? What kinds of treatments do you normally recommend for your AD/HD patients?

Parent Involvement and Education

I mentioned earlier that I think one of the most important factors in the successful treatment of AD/HD in a child is parent education about the disorder. If you have an AD/HD child, you need to become an expert on AD/HD. Read everything you can, go to seminars and conferences, and go to parent support groups. The more you know, the better off your child will be. This could be the number-one factor in your child's success. To help get you started, there is an extensive list of books and websites in the "Resources" section. I would also suggest that you join CHADD. Its *Attention!* magazine is stocked full of great information for parents.

Also, parent training with a licensed therapist can be very helpful. The therapist will analyze the problems that the family is experiencing and will recommend areas of change. The therapist basically helps the family develop new and improved ways of doing things. There is no need to feel embarrassed about going to a therapist for assistance. Having an AD/HD child can be the ultimate challenge to your parenting skills. Clearly, you can't do it all alone. While your AD/HD specialist will provide guidance, a strong relationship with your school is also essential.

Teacher Involvement and Education

Basically, you need to think of the entire school staff as a team dedicated to your child's education and well-being. This includes the primary teacher, teacher's aides, principal, secretaries, special education teachers, school counselor, art teacher, music teacher, computer teacher, physical education teacher, playground aides, bus drivers, cooks, and custodial staff.

The primary teacher, of course, has the most contact with your child. If she is positive and supportive, she can help your child not only learn the required material but also develop a love of learning. If she is not kind and supportive, however, your child could learn to hate school and hate himself. Your child's teacher can also set up various incentive activities for your child, such as star charts, point systems, or daily report cards. The primary teacher will also arrange for the individualized education plan to be implemented.

But your child doesn't just depend on his or her primary teacher. Many other people help educate your child throughout the school day.

Teacher's aides help with all the classroom stuff. They help tutor your child, help him with special projects, and help supervise him on field trips. The principal sets the atmosphere and the environment for the school. Is it a positive, loving, nourishing environment? The principal also takes part in special evaluations such as the IEP. Secretaries are also a big part of your child's education. They are the ones you call when your child is going to

be out for a doctor appointment or when your child is sick. They are frequently the ones who monitor the medications. Often, you have the most
contact with the school secretaries! Playground aides see the problems;
they see the fights; they see when a child doesn't have friends. You might
think that your child is doing well socially, but they see her sit every day
on the swings by herself. The school counselor can help your child with
problems she might have at school, as well as working on improving social
skills and organizing school support groups.

Is your child not gaining weight the way she should? Ask the cooks and
lunch monitors. They often can tell you what foods the children will eat
and what foods they won't touch. Is your child eating, or just talking? Is
she running out of time to finish her meal? Is your child having problems
with teasing or with a bully on the bus? Ask the bus driver. Your child forgot his book? The custodian can unlock the door so he can get it.

Your secondary teachers can also make or break your child. Does your
child have artistic ability? A good art teacher will recognize and encourage
this. Or does she see only the messes? A good music teacher may see the
hyperactivity as a benefit. These children often are stage pros! The list goes
on and on with these secondary teachers. Often, AD/HD children can
find ways that they can excel through music, art, and sports.

I can't tell you how important it is to have a supportive educational
team. If your school is not supportive, move your child to a different
school. Send your child to a private school if you think that would help. If
you need to, move to a different neighborhood. Your child should be a
major priority in your life. His education, happiness, and well-being should
be at the top of your list. Do everything you can to provide these things
for your child.

AD/HD Child Involvement and Education

It is all well and good to have a top-notch specialist, read all the AD/
HD books in the world, and be best friends with the school staff, but if
your child is left out of his or her treatment, it just won't work as well.

Treatment is not something we are doing to the child in order to cure
her and make her okay. Even if your child is preschool age, she needs a
voice and needs to be involved in her treatment process. This is so important! She needs to know why she is taking medication. She can also help

you monitor any side effects that could occur, as well as helping determine the optimum dosage level for her. Being aware and involved in the process can also help her with feelings of worthlessness and failure that are common among AD/HD children. If she doesn't know she has AD/HD, she might think she is a bad person or a failure. When she becomes an adult, her entire treatment process—including any therapy, coaching, or medication needed—will be her decision.

Remember, everyone has something. This is his something. We are working with him to find ways to help him cope with the disorder, to find ways that he can excel, and also to help him live a happy and productive life. We aren't curing him. We aren't fixing him. We are helping him find "tools" to help him build a well-constructed, strong life. A builder without any tools will have a very difficult time building anything.

SECOND LAYER

Okay, you have a top-notch doctor and you have educated yourself on AD/HD, developed a strong relationship with the school, and included your child in his treatment process. What else can be done?

Counseling

Some people are embarrassed about getting counseling. Don't be. AD/HD is way beyond our parenting skills. It is way beyond what most children can handle as well. We all can use help and guidance. It is a sign of strength, not weakness, to ask for help.

Individual counseling can help the AD/HD child with feelings of inadequacy, sadness, depression, and loneliness. A counselor will work with the child on specific social incidents. What happened? How did it make him feel? What options does he have in future incidents? Perhaps your child is embarrassed about his AD/HD or feels that he is alone and different. Support groups are a great way for a child to connect with other AD/HD children. And it's fun too. It also helps parents to connect and talk about their experiences. CHADD sponsors support groups around the United States. Contact them for a support group in your area.

One of area of counseling that you might not have considered is family counseling. Sometimes having an AD/HD child or two can upset the family balance. A hyperactive child often needs a great deal of attention, causing other children to feel neglected or left out. Family counseling can help the whole family work through issues such as household responsibilities, disagreements, and aggression between peers. Marriage counseling is also helpful to parents who are experiencing conflict in their marriage over how to handle the disorder. Let's face it: relationships are challenging enough. AD/HD is a difficult disorder. When you add the difficulties AD/HD causes to problems couples face, it can become pretty messy. You owe it to yourself, your partner, your AD/HD child, and your other children to try to work things out.

Academic Modifications

In addition to counseling, academic modifications can be a real benefit to AD/HD students and their teachers. There are numerous modifications that can be made. Special seating arrangements are very helpful for AD/HD children: they should be seated at the front of the classroom—near the blackboard and near the teacher's desk. When an AD/HD child sits near the front, the teacher can more easily monitor the child's off-task behavior. The teacher might have to redirect the child (such as a hand on the shoulder) often during the day. Sitting at the front of the classroom makes staying on task easier for the child as well. Also, the AD/HD student should be seated next to a mature, studious child—never next to the class clown. The other child can serve as a role model and act as a mentor. (In one of Theresa's classes, her "partner" would often help redirect her—"You need to put your book away" or "We're on page 27.") Some schools even have mentor programs where they partner an older child with a younger child. These programs are very valuable in helping AD/HD students.

There are other modifications that often help AD/HD children stay on task. Desk cubbies and dividers help block distracting views in front and on the sides of students so an AD/HD child can concentrate on his work. Some schools have the students make their own three-sided desk dividers out of cardboard and decorate them. And for older students, mechanical aides such as a laptop computer, word processor, or tape recorder can be invaluable. Fidgets and weighted vests are helpful items for hyperactivity.

Fidgets are stretchy balls or figures that a hyperactive child can manipulate. These objects help the child release unwanted energy during quiet periods. And weighted vests also help the child manage his energy levels appropriately.

Planners and accordion pocket organizers are a must. A daily planner should have an area for each subject. The child can write the assignment down and list the materials needed and the date the project is due. The parent can then see the homework assignment and initial it after it has been completed. The accordion organizer should have at least six pockets. Each pocket should be labeled with a different subject—for example, "spelling" or "math." In each pocket is a different-colored folder—for example, red for spelling and blue for math. Papers to go home should be placed in the left side of the folder and all papers to be returned to school in the right side of the folder. For example, all homework and study papers for science should be placed in the left side of the green folder and the folder placed in the science pocket. After the assignment has been completed, the homework should be placed in the right side of the green folder and returned to the science pocket. If different-colored folders, a pocket organizer, and a planner are used, all homework should come home with the child every night.

Tests can be overwhelming for an AD/HD student and sometimes do not accurately assess what they know! Testing accommodations can be made. AD/HD students often need additional time for tests. Sometimes an aide can help with the testing procedure by reading the questions aloud to the student. Removing the child to a quieter area for a test is also helpful.

Another helpful tool for the AD/HD child is resource-room participation. Some AD/HD children test lower in certain areas and will benefit by participating in a resource room for that subject—for example, being included in a special reading or math group. Small class size and one-on-one tutoring with a specialist in a weak area can be very helpful. One thing you can do as a parent is to ask your school if they have extra subject books for your child's class. You can either check these extra books out for the year or buy an extra set. If there is an extra set at home, you won't spend so much time running back and forth to school to retrieve missing items.

Of course, the value of having an advocate in the classroom and on field trips cannot be overstated. If a classroom aide is available, he or she can be a wonderful benefit to both the student and the teacher. (Theresa calls Mrs. Baxter, the aide in her classroom, her second mother.) Also, an adult should supervise the AD/HD child one-on-one for all field trips. Field trips can be fun and informative. They can also put an AD/HD child on overload. The child might run out into traffic, break a museum piece, or (as in our case) wander away from the group. One-on-one supervision is essential.

Occupational and Alternative Therapy Programs

Besides counseling and academic modifications, there are numerous occupational and alternative therapy programs that can help your child.

Sports and exercise are essential, not only for good health but also to help the AD/HD individual manage stress and excess energy. A few helpful sports are gymnastics, fencing, soccer, baseball, tennis, golf, volleyball, running, bicycling, shooting hoops, skating, surfing, skateboarding, tae kwon do, judo, and karate. I personally believe that AD/HD children should be involved in a sporting activity that is based more around individual participation—such as tennis, golf, running, and gymnastics—than a sport based on team participation. Sports that revolve around the entire team's winning or losing can put too much pressure on a child already stressed by failure. For example, if you miss catching a ball in baseball, your entire team could lose because of your failure. When one child's error causes a whole team and sometimes the coach to yell and scream at a child for failing, I believe, this does more harm than good to a child's self-esteem. I think that AD/HD children are best served by participating in a sport that is based more on individual performance rather than team performance. AD/HD children can still be part of a team and experience the benefits of being a part of a group, while avoiding some of the negative pressures involved with playing a sport.

Again, the Wilbarger Protocol for Deep Touch Pressure for children with sensory issues can be extremely helpful. This program helps them grow accustomed to touch. Also, art therapy (including painting, sculpture, and drawing cartoons) and music therapy (singing, dance, and playing an instrument) can be lifesavers for an AD/HD individual. Often AD/HD children excel in these areas. Relaxation therapies, including yoga and massage, are great stress reducers. Yoga can help an AD/HD individual with self-discipline and focus. Massage helps those with AD/HD to unwind.

Other occupational therapies that can be helpful include techniques to reduce activity level and improve concentration. One of the hospitals in our city has an occupational therapy program called the Engine Program. In the program, therapists provide patients (whose engines are on high) with coping strategies. You can check with your local hospital or therapy center about programs for AD/HD children.

As you can see, there a number of great treatment options in this layer!

THIRD LAYER

We've talked about counseling, sports, and occupational and alternative therapies, but there is one important treatment we have yet to discuss: coaching.

Coaching

Coaching is different from counseling. Counseling talks about feelings and how to deal with problems of various sorts. Coaching is exactly that— coaching individuals on how to perform certain tasks or to develop a skill set. Just as an athletic coach teaches someone how to throw a baseball or dribble a basketball, coaching an AD/HD child is based on the assumption that the child needs *practice* in a certain area. This might include practicing how to be safe in a parking lot, developing study skills, practicing how close to stand to someone, or practicing how to solve a playground conflict. These skills can be taught and developed.

I have had a great deal of experience with coaching. My mother was my teacher. When my brother was diagnosed with autism, the experts suggested that he be institutionalized. My mother is a fighter. I call her the "unsinkable Molly Brown." She read everything she could about autism and then designed a program to help my brother. Every day, each of us had numerous 15-minute coaching sessions with my brother. These sessions might be about how to hug, how to greet someone new, or even how to shave. (I actually taught my brother how to shave. Every morning, he and I would lather our faces. He would shave with a blade and I without. We did this not just once but every day for a year. If I ever grow whiskers, I'll be in great shape!)

The coaching lessons can be found in Chapter 10. They are fun and usually fairly short. Many of the lessons will seem like games to your elementary-school child. Among the coaching lessons are The Inchworm, to help teach social distance; Messy Mouth, to help teach appropriate table manners; and Treasure Hunt, to help your AD/HD child learn to follow instructions.

Charts and Behavioral Modification

Also, part of the complete treatment program includes behavior-modification charts. Behavior-modification star or point charts are a must for AD/HD children. They can be used at home and at school. Basically, an AD/HD child can earn points or stars for a special privilege. At school, points can be redeemed for extra computer or reading time, a special lunch with the teacher, or a small token of some sort. At home, points can be redeemed for an allowance or a special activity, such as a trip to the zoo or beach. Positive reinforcement works well. What tokens or rewards do you think your child would like? Use your imagination! Examples of behavior-modification charts can be found in Appendix A.

FOURTH LAYER

The fourth and top layer includes a very important aspect of the complete treatment process:

Medication

Let me tell you a short story. A couple that I know have an AD/HD daughter, but she was only just diagnosed. These two people are the best parents I have ever seen. For years, they tried different things to help their daughter. They went to numerous parenting seminars and read hundreds of books on children. They brought along grandparents and other relatives to help supervise her during community activities. They volunteered in her class. Although these things helped, they still despaired. Their daughter seemed unable to concentrate in school and her grades were low even though she was very intelligent. Finally, they had her tested. She was diagnosed with AD/HD and put on medication. I spoke with the father recently about how the medication was working. "It's incredible," he told me with amazement on his face. "We can really see a huge difference when she is taking her medication. We forgot last weekend, and, wow, it was really difficult."

Let me put it another way: If your child had the medical disorder of nearsightedness, you would have her tested and would purchase eyeglasses. In that case, eyeglasses are a tool to help her see better. The same is true with AD/HD. It is a medical disorder, and the medication is a tool. It helps AD/HD children pay attention and manage their hyperactivity.

The importance of medication cannot be stated enough. Research has shown that AD/HD children experience a 75 to 90 percent improvement in AD/HD behaviors with medication. If the ophthalmologist told you that glasses would improve your child's vision by this amount, you wouldn't hesitate. And yet many don't like the idea of medication to treat AD/HD in children.

Medication can help calm hyperactivity and focus attention. It can improve behavior and handwriting. It can even lower the odds of your AD/HD child using drugs. With results like these, the answer is obvious. Medication is an essential part of the AD/HD pyramid. The results could be substantial.

10.

COACHING
ASSIGNMENTS

. . . .

We can give our AD/HD children medication to help them concentrate at school. Medication helps a great deal. But it doesn't cure the disorder. The AD/HD is still there. Your child's grades might improve and his messy handwriting become legible. But he still forgets to bring his homework home. He still gets right in people's faces and talks incessantly. AD/HD children often don't pick up on things, especially social skills, which other, non-AD/HD children naturally do. What helps is to directly and consciously teach skills to your AD/HD child. In order for them to be successful and happy, they need to be coached by a loving, knowledgeable, and patient individual.

Have you ever been talking to someone new who stands too close to you, invading your personal space? I'm sure that all of us have had that experience at one time or another. Generally, we take a step backward to correct the problem. In some cases, the person will then move back into our space. At that point, one might think, "What's wrong with her? Doesn't she know she's standing too close?" or "Didn't he notice that I moved away from him?" Often, we then avoid this person because we feel uncomfortable and wonder what's wrong.

As children, we generally pick up on these types of things naturally.

When a child gets in another child's face, they are pretty blunt about it. Children generally "tell it like it is." "Get out of my face" and "You're too close" are typical responses, maybe with a physical shove. Most children learn from these experiences and social cues.

AD/HD children often don't learn these skills. Because of their attention problems, they may overlook the body language of others and may even miss out on important social lessons when told directly. "Get out of my face" to them might mean it is okay to be physically close but not to be close to someone's face. So instead, they might tackle the person. Or "You're too close" might mean that you are too close right now, but in a few minutes, that would be okay. Also, because of the social problems AD/HD can cause, AD/HD children often overcompensate with their friends. They might be too affectionate because they want to make sure they keep this friend. They might be too clingy and too possessive. She remembers the year when no one would sit with her at lunch. Or he might turn into the class clown, mistakenly thinking that his wild behavior will get attention and keep the attention on him. AD/HD children rarely realize that these types of behaviors could be misinterpreted as odd or strange and could actually cause additional social problems.

Physical space and other types of skills need to be consciously taught and practiced. For example, a lesson on physical space issues with your child would include the following:

- What is a person's physical space?
- Did you know that the appropriate distance between two people varies by country, culture, and friendship/intimacy level? For example, average personal space for Americans is greater than for individuals who live in Japan. This might be because there are many more people living in Japan and there is less space available per person. They are used to living in close proximity with one another.
- Have your child measure three feet with a tape measure. You stand on the zero and have your child stand on the three-foot mark. Talk for a minute or two. Does it feel comfortable to talk at this distance?
- Have your child measure out six inches. Stand six inches apart. Does this feel comfortable? Why not?

- Have your child measure out ten feet. Stand ten feet apart. Ask your child about his day. Does this feel comfortable? Why not?
- Discuss and practice social distance with your child. How close should you stand to a friend? How close should you stand to someone you just met? How close can you stand to a family member or your parents?

You can really make this a fun lesson. You can do ridiculous things by marking out fifty feet and asking them what they want for dinner. Or you can talk at three inches apart, with her nose at your bellybutton. Or if your child is older, then maybe your nose is at his bellybutton! It can get really silly. It should be fun, and yet informative. This lesson consciously looks at and examines social distance. It allows your child to see on a tape measure how close he should be and to practice this skill.

The following skill sets are divided into six areas: general social skills, manners, sensory issues, school, friendships, and safety issues. Each skill set is short and should not last longer than 15 minutes. Don't overdo it. Practicing skill sets twice a week is plenty. You don't want your child to feel that this is just one other thing they have to do—one other thing at which they are failing. When practicing a skill, keep it light. Don't ever say, "This is something you have to learn," or "This is something you still can't do, so we have to practice it." Instead explain that you are going to work on some fun activities and some silly games. Tell him these activities help people make friends and do well in school and are things everyone should know. Don't tell your child that you are doing these skill sets because of his AD/HD or because he is having problems or because his behavior is odd. Keep it light. Keep it fun, nonthreatening, and gentle.

When you practice these skill sets, you should repeat each lesson at least once. Two to four times is a good number. If your child becomes bored with doing one particular lesson, wait a couple of months and try it again. After you feel your child has mastered the lesson, you don't need to repeat it. Don't force your child to keep doing a lesson. You don't want her to get angry and then refuse to do anything else. Also, you can do these skill sets in any order. In my opinion, however, it is best to practice them by category. For example, in the month of March you can practice the "manners" skill sets and then reward your child by taking her to a nice restaurant to practice some of the techniques she has learned. It doesn't have to be expensive, just somewhere where you sit down and are served— preferably somewhere without a drive-through window and "Mc" in front of all names of food items.

Good luck. Remember to be patient. If it's not a good day and your child doesn't seem receptive to the idea, let it go for the day and try again later in the week. These lessons will help your child. And these lessons are only a beginning. Perhaps there are other areas in which your child needs coaching. Or you might have some new ideas. Discuss your ideas with your AD/HD specialist. These coaching lessons are a good jumping-off place.

Keep in mind that coaching is not counseling. Coaching involves skill sets that can be strengthened and improved upon. You can coach your child. Counselors, teachers, social workers, and psychologists can coach as well. There are also certified coaches available to help work with your child.

For further information on coaching, you can contact the following resources:

- CHADD at (800) 233-4050 or www.chadd.org.
- International Coach Federation at (888) 423-3131 or www.coach federation.org. ICF is a professional organization of both personal and business coaches. It offers a coach referral service.
- American Coaching Association (ACA) at (610) 825-8572 or www .americoach.org. ACA coaches work primarily with individuals with disabilities, including AD/HD. The organization offers a directory of coaches who are members of ACA.

LESSONS

General Social Skills

Developing social skills can be a very difficult area for AD/HD children. The skills won't necessarily come automatically to them. They often don't pick up on social cues that people send out. They might not notice when someone backs away from them. They might not recognize when it is okay to touch someone and when it isn't. An AD/HD child or adult can send the wrong signal to someone by not maintaining eye contact. Unlike non-AD/HD children, AD/HD children must be consciously taught social skills.

The Inchworm	TOPIC	SKILL SET	MATERIALS NEEDED
	Social distance or physical space #1	Learn appropriate distances to stand from family members, friends, and other people	14 or more paper inchworms (see end of Appendix A)

- Talk about personal space with your child. What is a person's physical space? It is the empty space around you that you need to feel comfortable.
- Talk about your own personal space with your child. Are there times that you feel uncomfortable when people are too close to you? For example, do you like to sit in the middle of a crowded movie theater or on the end of a row?
- Have your child talk about his or her personal space. Are there times that he feels uncomfortable when people are too close to him? If so, what are these situations?
- Show your child the inchworms that you have prepared. Measure the inchworm. (It should be six inches long.)
- Have your child place two inchworms in a line (one foot). You stand at the end of the first inchworm and have your child stand at the end of the last inchworm. Talk for a minute. Does it feel comfortable to talk at this distance? Why or why not?

- Have your child lay fourteen inchworms (seven feet). Now stand apart from each other at opposite ends. Does this distance feel comfortable? Why or why not?
- Have your child lay out six inchworms (three feet) and again stand apart from each other at opposite ends. Ask your child about his day. Does this distance feel comfortable? Why or why not?
- Discuss and practice social distance with your child. How close should you stand to a friend? How close should you stand to someone you just met? How close can you stand to a family member or your parents?

The Eyes Have It

TOPIC	SKILL SET	MATERIALS NEEDED
Maintaining eye contact #1	Learn why maintaining eye contact is important and practice the skill	None

- What is eye contact? It means to look into someone's eyes while they are talking to you. Often, body movements, such as nodding your head and smiling, go along with eye contact. This lets the other person know that you are listening to them and that what they are saying is important to you.
- Explain to your child why maintaining eye contact is important for social relationships. What would a person think if you looked all around the room, rather than at them, while they were talking? Would they think that you were interested in what they said? Would they think you were bored with them? Talk to your child about what the other person might think or do if you don't maintain eye contact.
- Pretend that you are talking with someone or on a date. Have one person look all around the room while the other person is talking.

Then reverse roles. How did that make you feel? What were you thinking when the other person was doing this?

- Now talk again. This time maintain eye contact. Talk about what body movements go along with your conversation.

People Watching

TOPIC	SKILL SET	MATERIALS NEEDED
Body language	Analyzing eye contact and body language in others	This lesson takes place in a crowded restaurant.

- Take your child to a crowded restaurant or other public place where people sit or stand across from each other.
- Refresh your child's memory on what it means to maintain eye contact. Discuss briefly what body language is usually used in a conversation.
- Watch other people. Be careful not to point to them or draw attention to the fact that you are watching them. Also, you should be far enough away to not be able to hear their conversation. You will be watching their body movements.
- Analyze different groups of people. Is she listening to him? Is she maintaining eye contact? What do her facial expressions say? What body language is she using? What is this couple's relationship? Are they in love? Are they friends? Do they not know each other?
- End the lesson. Enjoy a dessert and practice your own eye contact and body language together.

The Staring Contest

TOPIC	SKILL SET	MATERIALS NEEDED
Maintaining eye contact #2	Practice maintaining eye contact	None

- Did you ever have a "staring contest" with someone when you were a child? With a staring contest, each person looks into the other's eyes without looking away. You try not to laugh.
- Explain the rules of the game with your child. Have a staring contest.

She Loves Me,	TOPIC	SKILL SET	MATERIALS NEEDED
She Loves Me			
Not	Affection toward others	Learn to display appropriate levels of affection and friendship toward others	None

- Talk to your child about affection. What is affection?
- Whom do we show affection toward? Do we show affection toward our parents? How about brothers and sisters? What about our friends? Do we kiss the mailman? Do we hug the grocer? That's silly, isn't it?
- Talk about affection. What kinds of affection are appropriate? When is it okay to hug a friend? When is it not okay? When should we touch other people? Discuss different scenarios. How can you appropriately display affection toward others? What are some other ideas? (smiling, waving, nodding, saying something nice, etc.)

The Class	TOPIC	SKILL SET	MATERIALS NEEDED
Clown	Acting silly (class clown)	Distinguish when to do funny things and when to refrain	Puppets or dolls

- Pretend that the puppets or dolls are in a classroom. One doll is the teacher. Another doll is the class clown. Other dolls are students.
- Take turns operating the teacher puppet. Take turns operating the class clown puppet. Take turns operating the other student puppets.
- What does the teacher do? What does the class clown do? What do the other students think? Do they laugh? Do they think he is going to get into trouble? What happens?
- Talk about the different scenarios. Was his behavior a good idea? What would be some places or times where his behavior would be appropriate?

Sound Waves

TOPIC	SKILL SET	MATERIALS NEEDED
Developing listening skills	Improve listening skills	Four glasses, water, spoon, pitcher

- Talk about how we hear. Explain that when something produces a sound, sound waves move through the air and reach our eardrums.
- Put out four glasses, a spoon, and a pitcher of water. Have your child gently tap on the glass while you pour the water into the glass. What happens? (The pitch will change.)
- Use all four glasses. Have your child fill the glasses to various levels. What happens with the different water levels?

Do You Need Two Ears?

TOPIC	SKILL SET	MATERIALS NEEDED
Developing listening skills #2	Improve listening skills	Blindfold, musical instrument, chair

- Ask your child if having two ears helps with hearing. Would having one ear be okay? Is there any difference?
- Blindfold your child and have him sit in a chair.
- Quietly play the instrument three times (if you don't have one, bang gently on a pan). Have your child point in the direction of the sound. Walk to a different location and repeat. Repeat again.
- Now have your child plug one ear with his finger. Do the exercise again three times.
- Have your child take the blindfold off. How did he do? Most people will do better with both ears. This is because two ears help us hear direction.
- Switch spots. Have your child play the instrument and you guess.
- Other siblings might enjoy doing this also. They will also get a kick out of the mess-ups.

The Telephone Game	TOPIC	SKILL SET	MATERIALS NEEDED
	Developing listening skills #3	Improve listening skills	Five or more people, and paper, pen, or pencil

- Did you ever play the game Telephone when you were a child? Have the group of people sit in a circle. Have one person write down a phrase on a piece of paper, fold it, and hold it in her hand. Then she whispers the phrase to the person next to her. That person whispers the same phrase to the next person and so forth until the phrase is completely around the circle. The phrase may not be repeated.
- How did the last person do? Did he get it right or was it completely messed up?
- Try it again with a new leader.

Manners

Manners are important for adult life. Having appropriate manner skills might make a difference in a job interview or on a date. A lack of good manners can also be dangerous. Consider examples you might have heard about road rage incidents, someone stealing a parking space, or a fight at a department store over an item. Good manners must be practiced over and over with an AD/HD child. (There are a lot of non-AD/HD children and adults alike who could use a few refresher courses!)

Doors, Doors, Doors

TOPIC	SKILL SET	MATERIALS NEEDED
Opening doors #1	Learning how to use good manners and be polite	Different doors

- Did you realize that there are different ways to open doors for other people? Let me give you a few examples: (1) Open the door, stand back, and hold the door while the next person goes through it. (2) Open the door, go through it yourself, then turn around and hold the door behind you with one hand so the other person can "catch" the door before it falls. Also, other factors that should be taken into consideration include (1) the distance the next person is from you, (2) the heaviness of the door, (3) whether the door opens in or out, (4) whether the person is elderly or disabled in any way, (5) if the person is carrying an object. As you can see, this is not just a simple skill.
- Go to a shopping mall where there are numerous doors of different kinds. Practice having your child open the door for you. Switch and you open the door for your child. Practice saying, "Thank you."

Here, Let Me

TOPIC	SKILL SET	MATERIALS NEEDED
Opening doors #3	Learning how to use good manners and be polite	Different doors

- This is where it gets a little complicated. Talk with your child about different situations. For example, if someone is in a wheelchair, always open the door for him or her and wait for the person to go through before you do. Talk about other situations. For example, how far does a person have to be behind you for you to hold the door for them? A few feet? Or a hundred feet? Obviously, if the person is clear across the parking lot headed toward the store, there is no reason to stand there and wait. Practice different scenarios with your child.

	TOPIC	SKILL SET	MATERIALS NEEDED
Don't Cut!	Social distance while standing in line	Learn appropriate distances to stand from other people while standing in a line	One or two other people

- Talk about the lunch line at your child's school. What happens in the lunch line? Do people cut? How does this make you feel? Do they squeeze between two people? Do they push? What should they be doing? Do they race to the line to get in front of other people?
- Pretend you are at lunch. Have your child and the other people stand in line.
- You will be doing a little role-playing here. You pretend to be the disrespectful child. You push in between the other people. Talk about how that makes everyone feel. Take turns being the disrespectful child.
- Now practice getting into line. Practice walking. Practice the appropriate social distance to stand from the other people in line. How is it going?

Being a Lady
or Gentleman

TOPIC	SKILL SET	MATERIALS NEEDED
Table manners #1	Learn to use a fork, spoon, and knife appropriately	Plate, fork, knife, spoon, and food item

- A very important skill for adults is to have the proper table manners. Children often don't and must be taught. AD/HD children are even slower to learn the proper etiquette to use. They stuff their mouths, talk with food in their mouths, use the wrong utensils, jump up from the table, and so on. Each of these lessons deals with one skill. At the end of the lessons, take your child to a nice restaurant. It doesn't have to be expensive, just somewhere with napkins and silverware and where someone serves you.

- Tell your child that you are working on using a knife and fork today. Put a food item on the plate and practice the proper way to hold a fork and the proper way to use the knife and fork together. Start with an easy food item (like waffles, which won't move and are easy to cut). For subsequent lessons, try a challenge. Try cutting up blueberries or grapes. Have fun!

Yuck!

TOPIC	SKILL SET	MATERIALS NEEDED
Table manners #2	Learn how to carry on a conversation while eating	Plate, fork, knife, spoon, and food item

- Prepare a snack for your child that requires utensils. Explain the lesson. You will be eating and talking about his school day.
- Explain that he is not to talk with food in his mouth. Review the wrong way to do it. Talk with your mouth wide open with food. Have him do it. Isn't it disgusting?
- Then practice the skill while conversing and eating.

Messy Mouth

TOPIC	SKILL SET	MATERIALS NEEDED
Table manners #3	Learn how to use a napkin	Plate, fork, knife, spoon, napkin, glass, milk, and messy food item

- Prepare a glass of milk and a messy snack (such as pudding, yogurt, ice cream, etc.) for your child. Explain the lesson to your child. You will be learning how and when to use a napkin.
- First of all, do it the wrong way. Take a big drink of milk and let it get all over your mouth. Then take a bite of the messy food and keep eating. Get food all over your mouth. Smile. Have your child do the same.
- Then do it the right way. Show your child how to put your napkin on your lap. Show your child how to use the napkin appropriately. Have a nice time.

What Is a Good Sport?

TOPIC	SKILL SET	MATERIALS NEEDED
Good sportsmanship	Being a good sport	Go to a sporting event.

- Go to a sporting event with your child. This could be a professional game or just a neighborhood soccer game. Watch other people. Point out (not literally but by discussing it) people who are exhibiting good sportsmanship. Is there anyone who is being a bad sport? Why? How does his or her behavior make you feel? How do you think it makes the players feel?
- When one team or player loses, what does he do? Is he a good sport about losing? What would you do in his situation?

Are You a Polite Winner and a Good Loser?	TOPIC	SKILL SET	MATERIALS NEEDED
	Being a polite winner and a good loser	Being a good sport	Checkers or other board game

- Play a short game with your child (one you can play a couple of times in 15 to 30 minutes). Explain that you are going to practice being a polite winner and a good loser.
- Review with your child what it means to be a polite winner. For example, saying, "You played very well" or "I enjoyed playing with you." Can she think of any other polite things to say?
- What does it mean to be a rude winner? For example, "Uh-huh, uh-huh, I skunked you." Can your child think of any other rude things people have said to her when they have won a game? How did that make her feel?
- Practice playing the game. Practice being a polite winner and a good loser.

Taking Turns	TOPIC	SKILL SET	MATERIALS NEEDED
	Taking turns	Learning to be patient and take turns	Any game or activity that requires taking turns

- Prepare a game that requires taking turns for you and your child to play—for example, marbles or hopscotch. Explain that for a game to be fun, everyone needs to be patient and wait his or her turn.
- Talk about a time when someone didn't take turns. How did that make your child feel? Was the game any fun?
- Tell your child that you are going to act like a rude child at first. Be impatient and rude. Say things like, "Come on, I want to go!" Or "Hurry up, you're taking too long!" Have your child explain to you what you did wrong. Redo it and behave appropriately.
- Play the game again. Have your child behave appropriately. Compliment him each time he is patient and waits his turn. Compliment him for doing a good job.

The Thermometer	TOPIC	SKILL SET	MATERIALS NEEDED
	Anger management	Learning to constructively manage and control anger	Paper, pencil, crayons, markers

- Talk about things that make you angry with your child. Explain what you do to control that anger.
- Talk about things that make your child angry. Ask him what he does to control his anger.
- Talk about scenarios. What different things can you do when you are angry? (Examples: punch a pillow, run around the block, take deep breaths, etc.) What ideas can the two of you come up with?
- Draw a picture of two thermometers on a piece of paper—one cool and one hot. Talk about what things go in which reading. What are some things that make you mad? What can you do to bring that thermometer down?

Sensory Issues

Problems with sensory issues, such as a child's refusing to wear snow-pants or any clothing with zippers, can be helped with occupational therapy techniques. Some of these lessons can be practiced at home. A visit to an occupational therapist is also recommended for an AD/HD child with sensory difficulties.

Let's Dress Up!

TOPIC	SKILL SET	MATERIALS NEEDED
Tactile defen-siveness #1	Getting used to various clothing	Old clothes or costumes

- Get out some costumes or older clothes that you and your spouse have. Tell your child that you are going to play dress-up or have a fashion show.
- Try on the various clothes. Try to include different items and textures. Take pictures of some of the best or funniest outfits.

Messy Play

TOPIC	SKILL SET	MATERIALS NEEDED
Tactile defen-siveness #2	Getting used to messy textures	Bowl, messy food, other items as needed

- The idea with this activity is to allow your child opportunities to experience different textures on her skin. For example, you can make instant pudding and eat it with your fingers. You can use Play-Doh and make various objects. You can finger-paint. You can plant flowers in the spring with your child, or prepare a small garden.
- Any of these ideas can help your child experience and adjust to different sensory issues.

How Strong Are You?	TOPIC	SKILL SET	MATERIALS NEEDED
	Heavy-work activities	Calms over-active child	As needed

- Occupational therapists tell us that heavy-work activities can serve to calm an overactive child. Heavy-work activities include climbing a tree, pushing a wheelbarrow, yard work, vacuuming, walking in deep snow, swimming, dancing, and raking leaves.
- Talk about the Incredible Hulk. The comic book character has appeared in a television show and now a cartoon and a movie. Tell your child that he is going to turn into the Incredible Hulk. Ask him to do a few activities that the Hulk might find easy (such as shoveling snow or pushing a vacuum). Your child can even growl!
- For further information on heavy-work activities to help calm your child, you might want to see an occupational therapist.

School Issues

School and home are where children spend most of their time. At school, they need to be able to listen, to stay on task, and to follow instructions. Failure to follow the rules can be monumental and include below-ability scores, repeated grade levels, peer problems, and low self-esteem. We can help our AD/HD children improve their listening skills, stay on task, and follow instructions. It won't come naturally but, again, must be practiced. The development of these skills is similar to the development of musical ability. A person might not have a great deal of natural musical ability, but the more she practices, the better she becomes at playing the piano. And who knows? She might turn out to be a concert pianist! Our children can do better in school by learning and practicing these basic skills.

Treasure Hunt	TOPIC	SKILL SET	MATERIALS NEEDED
	Following instructions	Improving ability to quickly and accurately follow instructions or directions	Small snack items, plastic sandwich bags

- This is a fun activity. Buy a small bag of candy, nuts, or pretzels. Open the bag and divide the amount into smaller plastic sandwich or snack bags. Hide the bags around your home. Remember where you put them!
- Tell your child that you are going on a treasure hunt but that she will have to remember the instructions.
- Give your child two instructions at first. For example, "Look under your pillow and in your backpack." Have the child follow the instructions. As your child improves at the treasure hunt, give her more tasks at one time. For example, "Look in the refrigerator, look on a kitchen stool, look in your slipper, and then look under your bed."
- This activity will help your child improve her memory skills and listening skills while following instructions.

Find the Secret Object	TOPIC	SKILL SET	MATERIALS NEEDED
	Weeding out distractions	Improving ability to sort out distractions while focusing on a desired object	*Where's Waldo?* book

- Obtain a copy of *Where's Waldo?* or a similar book where you search for a hidden object. You can buy it from a bookstore or borrow one from the library.
- Sit and look at a page or two with your child. Look for Waldo. Who can find Waldo first?
- After you have found Waldo, ask your child, "Was there anything on this page that fooled you? Was there anything that distracted you from finding him?" Talk about what other items looked like Waldo.

	TOPIC	SKILL SET	MATERIALS NEEDED
Ring the Bell	Transitioning #1	Improve ability to make smooth and quick transitions	Bell, 10 activities at home

- Tell your child that you are going to play a "transitioning" game. Give your child a list of ten fun activities (for example, playing jacks, coloring, skipping rope). When you ring a bell, the child must quickly stop what he is doing and start on the next activity. You can make this really fun by making some very fast transitions.

	TOPIC	SKILL SET	MATERIALS NEEDED
Drop the Needle	Transitioning #2	Improve ability to make smooth and quick transitions	Stereo, tape cassette, or record

- Play the old game of Drop the Needle. Have child dance or move to the music. When the music stops, she must freeze. Other children can play along with this game.

Friendships

Making and maintaining friendships can be a major problem area for many AD/HD children and could have lifelong consequences. Studies have shown that by preschool, AD/HD children are already having problems with friendships and peer interactions. This area should be a major source of emphasis when coaching your AD/HD child.

Will You Be My Friend?	TOPIC	SKILL SET	MATERIALS NEEDED
	Making new friends	Improve ability to meet new friends	Books on friendship

- Talk with your child about friendships. Ask your child what she does when she meets a new person. What are some different ways she can get to know a new person?
- Read a book on friendship with your child. For children ages four to twelve, I suggest:

  The Care and Keeping of Friends. Nadine Bernard Westcott. Middleton, WI: American Girl Library, 1996.

  Friends. Helme Heine. New York: Aladdin, 1997.

  Who Will Be My Friends? Syd Hoff. New York: HarperTrophy, 1985.

  A Friend Is Someone Who Likes You. Joan Walsh Anglund. Orlando, FL: Harcourt Children's Books, 1986.

Be an Author	TOPIC	SKILL SET	MATERIALS NEEDED
	Making new friends #2	Improve ability to meet and make new friends	Paper, pencil, crayons, or markers

- Tell your child that you are going to be doing a special book on how to make friends. Have your child write the story and illustrate it. Read it together after he is done. Ask him about the story.

The Trouble with Bullies	TOPIC	SKILL SET	MATERIALS NEEDED
	Problems with teasing	Writing scenarios to help your child prepare for any teasing	Paper and pencil

- Talk with your child about teasing. Tell him about a childhood problem you had with a bully. Tell him how you tried to solve the problem. Did your solution work or not?
- What were some other options you could have used? Have your child help you make a list of scenarios or options. Which ones listed, in your child's opinion and your opinion, are better? Why and why not? (For example, hitting the bully. Not a good option. He could get badly hurt. You could get beaten up and get in trouble.)
- Review the positive options with your child.

The Tire Swing	TOPIC	SKILL SET	MATERIALS NEEDED
	When you aren't included	Developing options to deal with friendship difficulties	None

- Ask your child about a time she felt she wasn't being included in a game or activity with her friends. How did she feel?
- Pretend that two of her friends are on the tire swing. There isn't room for her too. Besides, the tire swing makes her sick. What are her options? Might she (1) offer to push them, (2) ask them to join you on the slide in five minutes, (3) find someone else to play with, (4) play by herself for a while. Are there any other options that the two of you can think of? Which option does your child like the best?

Punch and Judy	TOPIC	SKILL SET	MATERIALS NEEDED
	Disagreements with friends	Writing scenarios to help your child successfully resolve conflicts with her peers	Puppets or dolls

- Tell your child that the puppets are going to have a disagreement. Explain that you are going to try to find positive ways to work out the problems.
- Role-play with the puppets. Have one of the puppets get mad at the other puppet. Why is he angry? What can the other puppet do about

it? (For example, apologize, ask what is wrong, or try to make amends for what he has done.)

Personal Grooming

AD/HD children need extra practice on developing personal grooming habits. An AD/HD child might stick a toothbrush in her mouth for a few seconds and think that she is done. He might wash only the very top of his head and never behind his ears. The AD/HD will make them want to zip through the task, not paying attention to whether or not teeth are clean or clothes wrinkled. As your AD/HD child matures, this can create problems for him socially.

	TOPIC	SKILL SET	MATERIALS NEEDED
Brushing Is Good	Brushing teeth	Learning proper hygiene	Toothbrush, cup of water, toothpaste, and fake costume teeth

Having clean teeth and gums is important, not only for social reasons but also for a person's overall health. Recent studies have shown that tooth and gum disease can contribute to the risk of heart attacks.

- Show your child the fake teeth. These can be Dracula fangs, hillbilly teeth, or just funny teeth. Review proper brushing and flossing techniques with your child. Have your child practice brushing the fake teeth. Have him practice brushing his own teeth.

	TOPIC	SKILL SET	MATERIALS NEEDED
How Fast Are You?	Getting dressed	Decreasing time needed to get ready for the day	Notepad, pencil, and stopwatch

Getting our children dressed for school each morning is a major chore. I have discovered a few techniques that you can try, to help eliminate some of the morning difficulties:

- Give your child 15 minutes to get dressed, hair and teeth brushed, and face washed in the morning. Set a timer. If he is ready within that amount of time, he earns his points or appointed allowance for that day.
- Have your child lay out her clothes the night before.
- Play Beat the Clock. Time your child putting on each item of clothing. For example, four seconds for the pants and three seconds for the shirt. Try to beat his "best" time for each item. You can do funny things with this too. One day, I exchanged my daughter's socks with her younger brother's socks. When the stopwatch started, she had major problems. "Hey! What's going on here?" She started giggling. We had a good laugh about that one. Another time, I exchanged her socks with her dad's socks. She figured that out pretty quickly. Her whole leg would practically fit inside one sock!
- If getting ready for school is a major battlefield in your house, give your child his pill as soon as he gets up. This will help him stay on task.

	TOPIC	SKILL SET	MATERIALS NEEDED
Mr. Pointy Head	Washing hair	Learning proper hygiene	Shampoo

- Use lots of shampoo on your child's hair and lather it up well. Create unique hairstyles. Make one point straight up; make two points on either side; make a curly shape. Look in the mirror and laugh. Have fun. Wash and rinse hair very well. Explain how to get the hair very clean.

Safety Issues

Safety is another area of major concern with an AD/HD child or teen. Studies have shown that those with AD/HD have more emergency room visits and automobile accidents. Your child's AD/HD could cause him to be distracted and not notice a car backing out. It could cause him to impulsively run out into the street. When you remind him, he might say, "Mom, I already know that!" He might be able to recite the safety rule back to you, but is he practicing it?

	TOPIC	SKILL SET	MATERIALS NEEDED
Look Both Ways	Safety in a parking lot	Traffic safety	Grocery store parking lot

A parking lot can be a very dangerous place, especially for an AD/HD child. There are cars pulling into parking spots and cars backing out. There are people with carts everywhere and a great deal of noise.

Here are just a couple of safety concerns that children should be aware of:

- Don't expect that a car will stop to let you cross the street. It might not.
- Don't walk down the middle of the street aisle. Stay to one side or the other, but don't walk too close to parked cars. They might start backing up. Four feet is a good distance.
- Never bend over to get something or tie your shoe in the parking lot.
- Don't cut between cars to get from one aisle to another.
- Never run in a parking lot.

- Go to a grocery or shopping mall parking lot with your child. Practice going in and out of the store. Practice each of the above techniques. Get a small snack or token while you are there.

Walk, Don't Walk	TOPIC	SKILL SET	MATERIALS NEEDED
	Crossing at a crosswalk	Traffic safety	Street corner

There are numerous issues to consider when crossing on a "walk" signal:

- Don't stand too close to the curb while you are waiting. You might be hit by a car.
- Even though the sign says "walk," you must look both ways to see that there are not any stray cars still coming.
- You must walk quickly, but not run across the street.
- You must be across the street before the "don't walk" signal comes on.
- Take a trip downtown. Park your car and take a little stroll. Practice crossing the street at the crosswalks. Practice standing back from the curb. Practice waiting for the "walk" signal. Practice looking both ways before crossing. Practice a quick, brisk walk.

CONCLUSION

I had an interesting conversation with Jenny the other day. She came to me and began talking about a girl at her school.

"Mom, I think she has AD/HD. She's really hyper and she gets into trouble a lot," Jenny said. I had met the girl and had thought the same thing at the time.

"I think so too," I told her. "But it's not up to us to diagnose her."

"Yeah, but I think meds would really help her," Jenny replied.

"I agree," I said. "All of that is up to her parents though. But I think you are right about it."

She hugged me and ran off. It's interesting to me that she is able to recognize AD/HD behaviors. This is because she is aware of her disorder, accepts it, and is learning to deal with it. Now she wants to help others with similar behaviors, the way she has been helped.

With medication and the multimodal treatment methods discussed in this book, there is hope. Those with AD/HD can live happy and productive lives.

Appendix A

SAMPLE INCENTIVE CHARTS

Use the pages that follow as sample charts that can be tailored to meet your child's needs and your parenting style. You'll find charts for home and school with both financial and other reward-based incentives. You can use stickers, a point system, even smiley faces to keep track of your child's progress throughout the week.

The Inchworm Pattern on page 143 can be used for the social skill game The Inchworm, mentioned in Chapter 10. Make as many photocopies as you'll need; color and cut out. Or have your child decorate the inchworms. Once the game is mastered, the inchworms can be a fun decoration for your child's bedroom—and a great reminder of the skill he or she has learned.

FINANCIAL Incentive Chart

A job description for:

_____

Week of _____

Good Job!

	SUN.	MON.	TUES.	WED.	THUR.	FRI.	SAT.
Get completely ready for school (____¢)							
Make bed after getting dressed (____¢)							
Clear and rinse dishes after meals (____¢)							
Pick up your room (before bedtime) (____¢)							
Be nice to your siblings (____¢)							
Do your homework (5:00–6:00) (____¢)							
BONUS Help put laundry away (____¢)							
TOTAL ____							

TOTAL AMOUNT EARNED THIS WEEK! _____

Good Job!

SPECIAL ITEM Incentive Chart

A job description for:

_____

| Week of _____ |

	SUN.	MON.	TUES.	WED.	THUR.	FRI.	SAT.
Get completely ready for school (____ pts.)							
Make bed after getting dressed (____ pts.)							
Clear and rinse dishes after meals (____ pts.)							
Pick up your room (before bedtime) (____ pts.)							
Be nice to your siblings (____ pts.)							
Do your homework (5:00–6:00) (____ pts.)							
BONUS Help put laundry away (____ pts.)							
TOTAL ____							

TOTAL ITEMS EARNED THIS WEEK! _____

_____ = _____ POINTS

Good Job!

MORNING Incentive Chart

A job description for:

_____

Week of _____

	SUN.	MON.	TUES.	WED.	THUR.	FRI.	SAT.
Get out of bed (____¢)							
Get dressed (in clean clothes that match) (____¢)							
Brush your hair (____¢)							
Brush your teeth (must pass inspection) (____¢)							
Wash your face and hands (____¢)							
Make your bed (____¢)							
Eat your breakfast (____¢)							
Take your medication (____¢)							
Get your backpack together (____¢)							
TOTAL ____							

TOTAL AMOUNT EARNED THIS WEEK! _____

Good Job!

SPECIAL SCHOOL Incentive Chart

A job description for:

_____

Week of _____

	SUN.	MON.	TUES.	WED.	THUR.	FRI.	SAT.
Turned in homework from previous night (___pts.)							
Stayed on task (___pts.)							
Listened to instructions (___pts.)							
Transitioned to next subject in a timely fashion (___pts.)							
Was nice to classmates (___pts.)							
Filled out homework log for the next day (___pts.)							
Kept desk neat (___pts.)							
Stayed in seat (___pts.)							
BONUS (Returned library books on time) (___pts.)							
TOTAL ___							

TOTAL AMOUNT EARNED THIS WEEK! _____

Homework Log

DATE	ASSIGNMENT	ITEMS NEEDED	DUE	COMPLETED

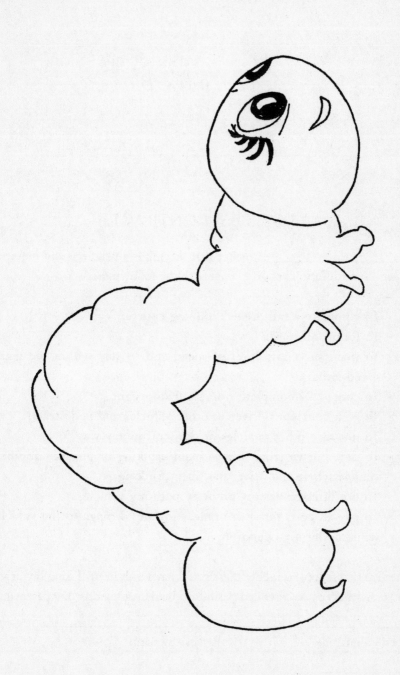

Appendix B

DRIVER'S CONTRACT

I, _____, realize that driving is a privilege and requires great responsibility. Therefore, I agree to the following:

- To complete a full driver's training course.
- To follow all traffic laws.
- To maintain a safe level of speed and to stay within the legal speed limit.
- To come to a complete stop at all stop signs.
- To be a courteous driver to other vehicles and pedestrians.
- To not race other vehicles or show off in any way.
- To never drive when I have been drinking or get into another vehicle where the driver has been drinking.
- To not litter or destroy property with my vehicle.
- To pay all costs (after insurance) for any damage to the vehicle while under my operation.

I realize that failure to follow these rules may result in my losing my driving privileges for an extended period (to be determined by my parents).

_____   _____
Teen's Signature   Parent's Signature

_____
Date

Appendix C

CHECKLIST FOR THE AD/HD PYRAMID

What to Expect About Testing

_____ Either you (the parents), a teacher, or a doctor becomes aware that there is a problem and identifies some of the AD/HD-type behaviors in your child.

_____ You (the parents), your child's school, or both parties decide that the child needs to be tested for AD/HD.

_____ You and your child visit the pediatrician to talk about the AD/HD-type behaviors and have your child tested to rule out other medical problems.

_____ You possibly receive a referral from your pediatrician to an AD/HD specialist, such as a psychiatrist, psychologist, or neurologist.

_____ You experience a long waiting period, from a few weeks to a few months, before your child is seen by the AD/HD specialist.

_____ You and your child attend a first meeting with the AD/HD specialist. This can last an hour or more.

_____ Both you and your child's schoolteachers will be asked to fill out numerous questionnaires.

_____ The AD/HD specialist will observe and test your child on two or more visits and evaluate the information.

What to Expect During and After Diagnosis

_____ The AD/HD specialist diagnoses your child with AD/HD (AD/HD-I, AD/HD-HI, or AD/HD-C type).

_____ The AD/HD specialist diagnoses any comorbid disorders in your AD/HD child, such as conduct disorder, Asperger's, or learning disabilities.

_____ The specialist discusses the various medication options with you and makes a recommendation.

_____ You are given a prescription for your child's AD/HD.

_____ You have your child try the medication for the first time on a weekend so you can watch for any changes or adverse reactions.

_____ You notify your child's teachers and day-care providers of the new medication. Ask them to watch for any changes or adverse reactions.

_____ You have frequent meetings at first with the specialist to monitor and adjust the medication type and dosage.

_____ You receive recommendations by the AD/HD specialist on other multimodal treatment suggestions.

_____ After your child's medication has been stabilized, you make plans to meet on a quarterly basis with the AD/HD specialist.

_____ If you are not happy with how treatment is progressing, you seek a second opinion by a different AD/HD specialist.

What Parents Can Do

_____ Join CHADD and start receiving *Attention!* magazine.

_____ Start reading everything you can about the disorder.

_____ Attend all scheduled parent/teacher conferences with the primary teacher, the resource-room teacher, and secondary teachers, such as art, music, and physical education.

_____ Help chaperone field trips with your child's class.

_____ Help music, art, and physical education teachers with their shows, field days, and activities.

_____ Attend support groups for parents of AD/HD children. For a list of support groups in your area, contact CHADD.

_____ Attend the sporting events, musical productions, art shows, and other activities in which your child participates—as many as you can.

_____ Twice a year, take your child on a "Special Day with Mom or Dad." (See page 67.)

_____ Spend quality time with your child whenever you can.

_____ Make sure not to neglect your other non-AD/HD children. Spend quality time with them as well.

_____ Arrange play dates with different children for your AD/HD child. Your child can work on developing her social skills. If she is experiencing social rejection in school, for example, this allows her alternatives.

_____ Listen to your child.

_____ Be involved in your child's life.

_____ Be consistent in your discipline. Be fair and consistent. Keep the rules simple. Post the rules in a prominent place in your home.

_____ Have a family meeting once a week to discuss weekly events and to work out problems.

_____ Pray, or meditate, for strength and patience every day.

_____ Offer lots of encouragement.

_____ Practice forgiveness and tolerance.

_____ Remember this word: *flexibility*.

_____ Give your child lots of love! And more love!

Helping Your Child Cope

_____ Tell your child about his or her AD/HD. Talk about the disorder and about ideas for treatment and medication. Read a children's book on AD/HD with your child or have your teen read a related book on his disorder.

_____ Enroll the child in an exercise or sport activity that he enjoys and is beneficial to him both physically and emotionally.

_____ Encourage the child to become involved in an activity or activities of her choice and interest. (For example: Girl Scouts of America, community theater, or 4–H.)

_____ Get involved with your child in community groups, such as attending a church or synagogue.

_____ Get involved in charity and environmental groups with your child. Help out at a soup kitchen with your child. Help clean up a river area. Help recycle. It helps them understand that someone, somewhere has it worse off than we do.

_____ Tell your AD/HD child, "Everyone has something." If they don't now, they will. This is your child's "something."

Special Issues for AD/HD Teens

_____ Encourage your teen not to drink or use drugs. Explain to them that AD/HD teens have a higher risk of substance abuse problems. In addition, don't drink and don't use drugs yourself. (You can make the statement, "We're in this together. I'm doing this for your well-being. If I'm asking you not to drink, then I won't either!")

_____ When your AD/HD teen reaches driving age, enroll him or her in a good driver's education class. Make sure they follow the guidelines in the driving contract in Appendix B.

_____ Work with your AD/HD teen to find an appropriate college or university. There are numerous books on this issue. For a list, see "Books" in the Resources section.

Helping Other People Understand AD/HD

_____ Supply your child's grandparents with information about the disorder.

_____ Invite grandparents, aunts, and uncles to your child's sporting events and music concerts. Grandparents are the best cheerleaders, even if your child comes in tenth.

What to Expect from Your Child's School

_____ You or the school can request testing for AD/HD or other disorders. This could be prior to the diagnosis or after the diagnosis by the specialist.

_____ After diagnosis, you and school members can meet to develop an individualized education plan (IEP) for the child.

_____ Meet twice a year with the committee to review the IEP and its success and to recommend any modifications needed.

_____ If possible, correspond weekly with your child's teacher on his academic and social progress, as well as any problems experienced.

_____ The school social worker or counselor can meet with your child to work with him or her on social issues or coaching lessons. Discuss this possibility with your child's teacher.

Implementation of Coaching Methods, Counseling, or Other Therapies

_____ Arrange for yourself, a counselor, a psychologist, an occupational therapist, or a social worker to start coaching techniques.

_____ If needed, you and the AD/HD specialist arrange occupational therapy for your child.

_____ If needed, you and the AD/HD specialist arrange individual therapy for your child.

_____ If needed, you and the AD/HD specialist arrange family counseling with a licensed practitioner.

_____ If needed, you and your spouse (or significant other) agree that marriage counseling is needed (or could be helpful).

_____ Consider other therapies as treatment for your child, such as music therapy, art therapy, massage.

Glossary

Abnormal: Anything outside of the normal range.

Academic Performance Rating Scale (APRS): A 19-item scale, for children in grades 1 through 6, that looks at a child's academic performance and accuracy.

ADA: See AMERICANS WITH DISABILITIES ACT.

ADD: See ATTENTION-DEFICIT DISORDER.

ADHD: See ATTENTION-DEFICIT/HYPERACTIVITY DISORDER.

AD/HD: See ATTENTION-DEFICIT/HYPERACTIVITY DISORDER.

AD/HD specialist: A physician who specializes in treating AD/HD.

Americans with Disabilities Act (ADA): A federal civil rights law established in 1992 that "prohibits discrimination against people with disabilities in everyday activities, such as buying an item at the store, going to the movies, enjoying a meal at a local restaurant, exercising at the health club, or having the car serviced at a local garage."

antidepressants: Medications used to treat depression include selective seratonin reuptake inhibitors (such as Paxil, Zoloft, Prozac, Celexa, and Lexapro), tricyclics (such as Elavil, Pamelor, Tofranil, and Sinequan), and others (such as Remeron, Effexor, and Valium).

anxiety disorder: A disorder characterized by disabling fear and apprehension.

Asperger's disorder: A mild form of autism.

assessment: Comparison of an individual's skill level against a norm or average.

attention: The ability to concentrate or focus on an activity.

attention-deficit disorder: Attention-deficit disorder involving inattention only. (See also ATTENTION-DEFICIT/HYPERACTIVITY DISORDER.)

attention-deficit/hyperactivity disorder (AD/HD or ADHD): A mental or behavioral disorder in which individuals experience abnormal levels of inattention and/or hyperactivity and impulsivity.

auditory sensitivities: Being overly sensitive to certain sounds and sound levels.

autism or autistic disorder: Disorder characterized by abnormal social skills, including difficulties interacting with other people, poor communication skills (both verbal and nonverbal), and odd, repetitive patterns of behavior (including rocking motions, spinning objects, etc.).

basal ganglia: Inner section of the brain. The basal ganglia help control attention levels, thought processes, and movement.

behavior modification: The use of positive and negative consequences to modify behavior.

blue baby: A condition in which a newborn baby receives an inadequate amount of oxygen, both during and shortly after the birthing process. This can be caused by the umbilical cord being around the child's neck or other birthing complications. Often the infant is motionless and blue in color. These infants often require emergency service.

booster pill: An additional, smaller dose of an AD/HD medication, usually taken later in the day, to help control AD/HD symptoms. These pills are often used to help an AD/HD child function during an important event.

Brethine: A medication used to treat asthma, as well as premature labor in pregnant women.

central nervous system (CNS): The brain and spinal cord.

cerebellum: Section of the brain found in the back of the head near the neck. The cerebellum is involved in higher thinking skills such as logic, time management, and reasoning skills. The midline vermis of the cerebellum, in particular (one of the smaller areas of the brain affecting children with AD/HD), helps control and modulate the brain's dopamine levels, as well as energy and locomotion levels.

child psychiatrist: A medical doctor who specializes in treating children with mental and emotional disorders.

Children's Attention Problems (CAP): this scale is a weekly scale used by teachers to help determine treatment outcome.

Children's Depression Inventory (CDI): This test looks for abnormal amounts of sadness or depression in a child.

chromosome: A strand of DNA within the nucleus of a cell that carries genes and transmits hereditary information.

classroom observation: Watching a child's behavior and functioning level in the classroom environment.

coaching: Assisting an individual in the development of social, safety, and daily living skills.

comorbid disorders: A different disorder that often goes along with or accompanies AD/HD. Examples of comorbid disorders include learning disabilities, obsessive-compulsive disorder, Asperger's disorder, conduct disorder, and anxiety disorders.

compensation: Behavioral techniques used to offset a problem or difficulty.

conduct disorder (CD): A disorder in which the individual is violent, hurts others, and destroys physical items.

consensus statement: This means that all listed parties agree. An example includes the 2002 International Consensus Statement on AD/HD.

controversy: Issue of intense disagreement.

cure: To restore health or completely correct a disorder.

depression: A feeling of sadness or despondency.

depressive disorder: A disorder where the individual is extremely depressed and sad. This disorder is characterized by eating too much or too little, problems sleeping, and thoughts of death or suicide.

diagnosis: The identification of the cause of a disease or disorder.

diagnostic guidelines: The primary guidelines or criteria for receiving a diagnosis of AD/HD are found in the American Psychiatric Association's *Diagnostic and Statistical Manual of Mental Disorders,* 4th edition (or *DSM-IV*).

Diagnostic Interview Schedule for Children (DISC): A test used to assess mood disorders in children.

disease: A pathological condition in the body as a result of an infection or virus, a genetic defect, or an environmental cause.

disorder: A problem or a condition within the body that is not in the normal range of function.

distractibility: The inability to weed out distractions.

distractions: Items that divert attention away from the item currently being focused upon.

dopamine: A neurotransmitter, or chemical found in the brain, that controls physical movement and attentiveness.

dopamine hypothesis: The scientific belief that problems with transportation of the neurotransmitter dopamine is partly responsible for attention-deficit/hyperactivity disorder.

dorsolateral prefrontal circuits: Dorsolateral means "back and both sides." Prefrontal is the lobe in the brain that controls higher functions.

dosage: Amount of medication prescribed.

downtime problems: Increase in inattention, hyperactivity, and impulsivity levels due to the first dosage wearing off and the second dosage not yet taking effect.

drug holiday: A break from medication use in AD/HD children (often on the weekends or over the summer).

DSM-IV (*Diagnostic and Statistical Manual of Mental Disorders,* 4th edition): Criteria from this diagnostic manual are the primary tool used to help evaluate an individual for AD/HD.

dyslexia: A reading disorder characterized by inverting and transposing letters and words.

dysthymic disorder: Chronic, long-lasting depression (lasting more than two years).

electroencephalogram (EEG): A machine that records electrical brain activity or brain waves.

FAPE (free appropriate public education): Two federal laws guarantee a free, appropriate public education for children. The first is civil rights law, Section 504 of the Rehabilitation Act of 1973. The second is an education law, Individuals with Disabilities Education Act (IDEA).

first-line medication: Drugs used as the first choice of treatment.

food allergy: An allergy to a food, such as strawberries or nuts. The allergy can be as simple as a small rash, or as dangerous as a systemic, life-threatening reaction.

generalized anxiety disorder (GAD): A disorder where the individual is extremely anxious or worried.

generic: A medication that does not have a brand name or trademark. The public generally thinks of generic drugs as costing less money than a brand-name product.

genes: A specific unit or section on a chromosome. Genes determine particular traits and characteristics.

genetic markers: Abnormalities on particular chromosomes that determine or indicate a disease or disorder. Scientists have discovered abnormalities on the following chromosome regions in those with AD/HD: 16p13, 17p11, and 5p13.

genomewide scan: A genetic scan that compares and contrasts genes between different groups of people. When scientists do a genomewide scan, they are looking for a linkage or similarities on particular chromosomes.

hyperactivity: The condition of being overly or excessively active.

hyperkinesis: An early term used for AD/HD. In Latin, this word means "superactive." In other Western countries, the term *hyperkinetic* is still used rather than AD/HD.

impulsivity: Acting on a sudden urge or impulse rather than thinking through the action rationally before acting.

inattention: Inability to stay on task or weed out distractions (a key symptom of AD/HD).

individualized education program (IEP): A list of specific skills that a child in a special education program will be taught. It is an agreement between the school and the family and is guaranteed under IDEA.

Individuals with Disabilities Education Act (IDEA): IDEA is an education law. To receive special education services under IDEA, a child must have "ADHD that results in a heightened alertness to stimuli in the classroom that limits alertness to academic tasks" and is "long-lasting (chronic) or have a substantial impact (acute)."

Iowa Conners' Teacher's Rating Scale: Based on the Conners' Teacher Rating Scale, this teacher report form compares AD/HD-type behavior with oppositional-defiant behavior.

learning disability: A disorder characterized by difficulties in reading, writing, or math despite normal or above-normal intelligence levels.

magnetic resonance imaging (MRI): A test that uses radio waves and magnetic fields to produce images of the body.

medical tests: Medical tests are either invasive or noninvasive procedures done to examine something in the body. This can include a blood test where the specialist is looking for a certain bacterium, an X-ray of a broken bone, or an MRI showing the presence of a brain tumor.

meltdown: Intense crying, screaming, or kicking by an AD/HD child. Often the cause or trigger of the meltdown cannot be identified.

minimal brain dysfunction (MBD): An older term originally used to refer to minor brain damage.

monoamine oxidase inhibitors (MAOI): An older classification of antidepressant drug seldom used today. MAOIs are normally used with adult patients.

multimodal management plan: A system of treatment for AD/HD involving medication, education, counseling, and coaching programs.

neuroimaging: Medical tests that take images or pictures of the brain. These include the MRI and CAT scan.

neurologist: A doctor of medicine who specializes in treating diseases and disorders of the central nervous system.

neurotransmitter: A chemical in the brain that transmits nerve impulses.

obsessive compulsive disorder (OCD): A type of anxiety disorder where the individual must repeat actions in order to overcome their distress.

oppositional defiant disorder (ODD): A behavior pattern in which the individual is defiant and aggressive.

orbitomedial prefrontal circuits: *Orbit* means eye. "Medial" means "pertaining to." This refers to the front section of the brain behind the eyes.

parent education: Education of parents about AD/HD. This is an ongoing process and is achieved by reading books and articles, visiting websites about the disorder, attending meetings and presentations about AD/HD, participating in teleconferences, and attending group support meetings.

pediatrician: A physician who specializes in the treatment of children's diseases and disorders.

Physicians' Desk Reference (PDR): A publication used by doctors, which gives pertinent information about medications.

prefrontal cortex: Right and left front lobes of the brain. The prefrontal cortex assists in analyzing social cues, controlling behaviors, sorting out distractions, sustaining and focusing attention, and controlling emotions, as well as assisting in short-term memory. The *right* prefrontal cortex helps us determine what to pay attention to and what to ignore.

premature delivery: Birth of an infant before 38 weeks.

proprioceptive: Relating to the joints.

psychiatrist: A doctor (M.D.) who specializes in diagnosing and treating mental and emotional disorders.

psychological tests: Questionnaires that score the individual against national averages. This includes psychological tests for AD/HD, intelligence, depression, compulsive behaviors, and schizophrenia.

psychologist: A Ph.D. who specializes in research, testing, and therapy of those with mental and emotional disorders.

Section 504: A federal civil rights law that prohibits schools (because they receive federal funds) from "discriminating against children with disabilities" and requires that they "provide disabled children with reasonable accommodations."

seizure: A sudden convulsion or spasm, often the result of epilepsy or another disorder.

selective norepinephrine reputake inhibitors (SNRIs): Prescription medications, some of which are approved to treat AD/HD. SNRIs inhibit the reuptake of norepinephrine.

selective serotonin reuptake inhibitor (SSRI): A type of antidepressant that stops the reuptake of serotonin in the brain and allows it to stay in the system longer.

sensory difficulties: Oversensitivity in any or all of three sensory areas (TACTILE, PROPRIOCEPTIVE, and VESTIBULAR).

separation anxiety disorder: A disorder where the individual experiences debilitating anxiety over leaving home or being separated from another individual.

SKAMP: A 10-item scale used to help identify and diagnosis AD/HD. This scale measures how well a child functions at school and at home.

sleep disorder: A disorder characterized by difficulty going to sleep or staying asleep.

sleep disorder clinic: A medical facility where specialists monitor and test for sleep-related difficulties and disorders.

SNAP-IV: A 26-item scale, based on the *DSM-IV* criteria, used to help diagnosis of AD/HD.

social skills: Proficiency in social situations.

support group: A group of people with the same disease, disorder, or disability, or a similar tragic event (or parents of an affected individual) who meet to discuss problems and solutions and offer guidance and support.

tactile: Relating to touch.

tactile defensiveness: Aversion or oversensitivity to certain textures or touch.

Test of Variable Attention (TOVA): A common psychological questionnaire used to help diagnosis of AD/HD.

tic disorder: Vocal tic disorders include behaviors such as throat clearing, snorting, sniffing, shouting, humming, and other odd vocalizations. Motor tics include eye blinking, facial grimaces, head jerking, and other odd physical movements.

Tourette's syndrome: A specific TIC DISORDER where the individual has involuntary body movements (such as head jerking or eye blinking), often accompanied by various vocal tics (including yelling, shouting, sniffing, etc.).

ventral frontal circuits: "Ventral" means lower. This refers to the lower, front section of the brain.

vestibular: Relating to movement.

Wechsler Intelligence Scale for Children, Revised (WISC-R): This scale tests intelligence levels against ability levels.

Wilbarger Protocol for Deep Touch Pressure: A program (developed by Dr. Wilbarger in 1991) that uses soft, surgical brushes and deep compression to help relieve anxiety and reduce sensory defensiveness.

Zung Self-Rating Depression Scale (SDS): A scale used for teens and adults that screens for depression by asking questions of the participant.

References

ALTERNATIVE THERAPIES

Chan, Eugenia. "The role of complementary and alternative medicine in Attention-Deficit/Hyperactivity Disorder." *Journal of Developmental & Behavioral Pediatrics,* February 2002: 37–45.

Chan, Eugenia; Leonard A. Rappaport; and Kathi J. Kemper. "Complementary and alternative therapies in childhood attention and hyperactivity problems." *Journal of Developmental & Behavioral Pediatrics,* February 2003: 4–8.

AUTISM, ASPERGER'S DISORDER, AND AD/HD

Gillberg, Christopher, and Linda De Souza. "Head circumference in autism, asperger syndrome, and ADHD: a comparative study." *Journal of the American Academy of Child and Adolescent Psychiatry,* January 2003: 115.

BIPOLAR DISORDER AND AD/HD

Sachs, Gary S.; Claudia F. Baldassano; Christine J. Truman; and Constance Guille. "Comorbidity of Attention-Deficit/Hyperactivity Disorder with Early- and Late-Onset Bipolar Disorder." *American Journal of Psychiatry,* March 2000: 466–68.

Tucker, Miriam E. "Test helps draw line between bipolar, ADHD." *Clinical Psychiatry News,* January 2004: 4.

BRAIN IMAGING STUDIES

Banaschewski, Tobias, et al. "Association of ADHD and conduct disorder: brain electrical evidence for the existence of a distinct subtype." *Journal of Child Psychology and Psychiatry and Allied Disciplines,* March 2003: 356–76.

Bastain, Theresa M., et al. "Cytogenetic abnormalities in attention-deficit/hyperactivity disorder." *Journal of the American Academy of Child and Adolescent Psychiatry,* July 2002: 806–10.

Castellanos, F. Xavier, et al. "Developmental trajectories of brain volume abnormalities in children and adolescents with Attention-deficit/hyperativity disorder." *Journal of the American Medical Association,* October 9, 2002: 1740–48.

Jensen, Eric. *Different Brains, Different Learners: How to Reach the Hard to Reach.* San Diego, CA: Brain Store, 2000.

Loo, Sandra K., et al. "Functional effects of the DAT1 polymorphism on EEG measures in ADHD." *Journal of the American Academy of Child and Adolescent Psychiatry,* August 2003: 986–93.

Sanjiv, Kumra. "Examining Brain Connectivity in ADHD." *Psychiatric Times,* January 1, 2004: 40.

Yeo, Ronald A., et al. "Proton magnetic resonance spectroscopy investigation of the right frontal lobe in children with attention-deficit/hyperactivity disorder." *Journal of the American Academy of Child and Adolescent Psychiatry,* March 2003: 303–10.

CONDUCT DISORDER AND AD/HD

Biederman, Joseph; Erik Mick; Stephen V. Faraone; and Melissa Burback. "Patterns of remission and symptom decline in conduct disorder: A four-year prospective study of an ADHD sample." *Journal of the American Academy of Child and Adolescent Psychiatry,* March 2001: 290–92.

FAMILY ISSUES

"ADHD parents." *Pediatric Nursing,* February 2004: 4.

Lougy, Richard, and David Rosenthal. *ADHD: A Survival Guide for Parents and Teachers.* Duarte, CA: Hope Press, 2002.

Bussing, Regina, et al. "Child temperament, ADHD, and caregiver strain: exploring relationships in an epidemiological sample." *Journal of the American Academy of Child and Adolescent Psychiatry,* February 2003: 184–92.

Edwards, Gwenyth, et al. "Parent-adolescent conflicts in teenagers with ADHD and ODD: The role of parental maladjustment." *Journal of Abnormal Child Psychology,* December 2001: 557–72.

Epstein, Jeffery N., et al. "Familial Aggregation of ADHD Characteristics." *Journal of Abnormal Child Psychology,* December 2000: 585–94.

Harrison, Christine, and Kate Sofronoff. "ADHD and parental psychological distress: role of demographics, child behavioral characteristics, and parental cognitions." *Journal of the American Academy of Child and Adolescent Psychiatry,* June 2002: 703–11.

Heininger, Janet E., and Sharon K. Weiss. *From Chaos to Calm: Effective Parenting for Challenging Children with ADHD and Other Behavioral Problems.* New York: Berkley Publishing Group, 2001.

Hinshaw, Stephen P., et al. "Family processes and treatment outcome in the MTA: Negative/ineffective parenting practices in relation to multimodal treatment." *Journal of Abnormal Child Psychology,* 2000: 555–60.

Hoza, Betsy, et al. "Parent Cognitions as Predictors of Child Treatment Response in Attention-deficit/Hyperactivity Disorder." *Journal of Abnormal Child Psychology,* December 2000: 569.

"Hyper Kids: What every parent needs to know about ADHD." *Prevention,* January 2004: 91.

Johnston, Charlotte, et al. "Responsiveness in interactions of mothers and sons with ADHD: Relations to maternal and child characteristics." *Journal of Abnormal Child Psychology,* February 2002: 77–88.

Johnston, Charlotte, et al. "Effects of stimulant medication treatment on mothers' and children's attributions for the behavior of children with attention-deficit hyperactivity disorder." *Journal of Abnormal Child Psychology,* August 2000: 371–73.

Landgraf, Jeanne M.; Michael Rich; and Leonard Rappaport. "Measuring quality of life in children with attention-deficit/hyperactivity disorder and their families: development and evaluation of a new tool." *Archives of Pediatrics & Adolescent Medicine,* April 2002: 384–91.

"Parents of ADHD patients need care, too." *Clinician Reviews,* March 2004: 40.

Stein, Martin T.; Lawrence Diller; and Roy Resnikoff. "ADHD, divorce, and parental disagreement about the diagnosis and treatment." *Journal of Developmental & Behavioral Pediatrics,* April 2001: 61–62.

Wells, Karen C., et al. "Parenting and family stress treatment outcomes in attention-deficit hyperactivity disorder (ADHD): an empirical analysis in the MTA study." *Journal of Abnormal Child Psychology,* December 2000: 543–48.

GENDER ISSUES

Abikoff, Howard B., et al. "Observed classroom behavior of children with ADHD: relationship to gender and comorbidity." *Journal of Abnormal Child Psychology,* August 2002: 349–59.

Biederman, Joseph, and Thomas J. Spencer. "Genetics of childhood disorders: XIX. ADHD, Part 3: Is ADHD a noradrenergic disorder?" *Journal of the American Academy of Child and Adolescent Psychiatry,* 2000: 1330–39.

Biederman, Joseph, et al. "Influence of gender on attention-deficit/hyperactivity disorder in children referred to a psychiatric clinic." *American Journal of Psychiatry,* January 2002: 36–42.

GENETICS

Barkley, Russell A. "Genetics of Childhood Disorders: XVII. ADHD, Part 1: The Executive Functions and ADHD." *Journal of the American Academy of Child and Adolescent Psychiatry,* August 2000: 1064–71.

Barr, Cathy L. "Genetics of childhood disorders: XXII. ADHD, Part 6: The dopamine D4 receptor gene." *Journal of the American Academy of Child and Adolescent Psychiatry*, January 2001: 118.

Faraone, Stephen V.; Alysa E. Doyle; Eric Mick; and Joseph Biederman. "Meta-analysis of the association between the 7-repeat allele of the dopamine [D.sub.4] receptor gene and attention-deficit hyperactivity disorder." *American Journal of Psychiatry*, July 2001: 1052.

Fisher, Simon E., et al. "A genomewide scan for loci involved in attention-deficit/hyperactivity disorder." *American Journal of Human Genetics*, May 2002: 1183–96.

Gainetdinov, Rauld R., and Marc G. Caron. "Genetics of childhood disorders: XXIV. ADHD, Part 8: Hyperdopaminergic mice as an animal model of ADHD." *Journal of the American Academy of Child and Adolescent Psychiatry*, March 2001: 380–82.

Langley, Kate, et al. "Association of the dopamine [D.sub.4] receptor gene 7-repeat allele with neuropsychological test performance of children with ADHD." *American Journal of Psychiatry*, January 2004: 133–48.

Lowe, Naomi, et al. "Joint analysis of the DRD5 marker concludes association with attention-deficit/hyperactivity disorder confined to the predominantly inattentive and combined subtypes." *American Journal of Human Genetics*, February 2004: 348–56.

Ogdie, Matthew N., et al. "A genomewide scan for attention-deficit/hyperactivity disorder in an extended sample: suggestive linkage." *American Journal of Human Genetics*, May 2003: 1268–79.

Smalley, Susan L., et al. "Genetic linkage of attention-deficit/hyperactivity disorder on chromosome 16p13, in a region implicated in autism." *American Journal of Human Genetics*, October 2002: 959–63.

Sunohara, G. A., et al. "Linkage of the dopamine [D.sub.4] receptor gene and attention-deficit/hyperactivity disorder." *Journal of Developmental & Behavioral Pediatrics*, June 2001: 205–7.

Wigg, Karen, et al. "Attention-deficit hyperactivity disorder and the gene for dopamine beta-hydroxylase." *American Journal of Psychiatry*, June 2002: 1046–48.

GIRLS AND AD/HD

Biederman, Joseph, et al. "Efficacy of atomoxetine versus placebo in school-age girls with attention-deficit/hyperactivity disorder." *Pediatrics*, December 2002: 1242–43.

Blachman, Dara R., and Stephen P. Hinshaw. "Patterns of friendship among girls with and without attention-deficit/hyperactivity disorder." *Journal of Abnormal Child Psychology*, December 2002: 625–40.

Castellanos, F. Xavier, et al. "Quantitative brain magnetic resonance imaging in girls with attention-deficit/hyperactivity disorder." *Archives of General Psychiatry*, March 2001: 289–91.

Castellanos, F. Xavier, et al. "Executive function oculomotor tasks in girls with ADHD." *Journal of the American Academy of Child and Adolescent Psychiatry*, May 2000: 644–50.

Farone, Stephen V., et al. "Family study of girls with attention-deficit hyperactivity disorder." *American Journal of Psychiatry*, July 2000: 1077–83.

Greene, Ross W., et al. "Social impairment in girls with ADHD: patterns, gender comparisons, and correlates." *Journal of the American Academy of Child and Adolescent Psychiatry*, June 2001: 704–9.

Hinshaw, Stephen P., et al. "Preadolescent girls with attention-deficit/hyperactivity disorder: II. Neuropsychological performance in relation to subtypes and individual classification." *Journal of Consulting and Clinical Psychology,* October 2002: 1099–1112.

Hinshaw, Stephen P. "Preadolescent girls with attention-deficit/hyperactivity disorder: I. Background characteristics, comorbidity, cognitive and social functioning, and parenting practices." *Journal of Consulting and Clinical Psychology,* October 2002: 1086–98.

Kato, Pamela M.; Mary L. Nichols; Amy S. Kerivan; and Lynne C. Huffman. "Identifying characteristics of older and younger females with attention-deficit/hyperactivity disorder." *Journal of Developmental & Behavioral Pediatrics,* October 2001: 306–15.

Nadeau, Kathleen; Patricia Quinn; and Ellen Littman. *Understanding Girls with Attention-Deficit/Hyperactivity Disorder.* Silver Spring, MD: Advantage Books, 2000.

HEALTH CARE COSTS

Chan, Eugenia; Chunliu Zhan; and Charles J. Homer. "Health care use and costs for children with attention-deficit/hyperactivity disorder: national estimates from the Medical Expenditure Panel Survey." *Archives of Pediatrics & Adolescent Medicine,* May 2002: 504–11.

Guevara, James, et al. "Utilization and cost of health care services for children with attention-deficit/hyperactivity disorder." *Pediatrics,* July 2001: 71–78.

Leibson, Cynthia L., et al. "Use and costs of medical care for children and adolescents with and without attention-deficit/hyperactivity disorder." *Journal of the American Medical Association,* January 3, 2001: 60–66.

Sandler, Adrian D. "Attention-deficit/hyperactivity disorder: health care costs." *Journal of Developmental & Behavioral Pediatrics,* October 2002: 391.

LEARNING DISABILITIES AND AD/HD

Aaron, P. G., et al. "Separating genuine cases of reading disability from reading deficits caused by predominantly inattentive ADHD behavior." *Journal of Learning Disabilities,* September–October 2002: 425–36.

Doyle, Alysa E.; Stephen V. Faraone; Emily P. DuPre; and Joseph Biederman. "Separating attention-deficit/hyperactivity disorder and learning disabilities in girls: a familial risk analysis." *American Journal of Psychiatry,* October 2001: 1666–72.

Greenbaum, Judith, Alice Beresin (illustrator); and Geraldine Ponte Markel. *Helping Adolescents with ADHD and Learning Disabilities: Ready-to-Use Tips, Techniques and Checklists for School Success.* Hoboken, NJ: Jossey-Bass, 2001.

Rae, Caroline; Martin A. Lee; and Ruth M. Dixon. "Metabolic abnormalities in developmental dyslexia detected by 1H magnetic resonance spectroscopy." *The Lancet,* June 20, 1998: 1849.

Weiler, Michael David; Jane Holmes Bernstein; David Bellinger; and Deborah P. Waber. "Information processing deficits in children with attention-deficit/hyperactivity disorder, inattentive type, and children with reading disability." *Journal of Learning Disabilities,* September–October 2002: 448–61.

Willcutt, Erik G., et al. "A comparison of the cognitive deficits in reading disability and attention-deficit/hyperactivity disorder." *Journal of Abnormal Psychology,* 2001: 157.

MATERNAL SMOKING

Linnet, Karen Markussen, et al. "Maternal lifestyle factors in pregnancy risk of attention-deficit/hyperactivity disorder and associated behaviors: review of the current evidence." *American Journal of Psychiatry,* June 2003: 1028–40.

Mick, Eric, et al. "Case-control study of attention-deficit/hyperactivity disorder and maternal smoking, alcohol use, and drug use during pregnancy." *Journal of the American Academy of Child and Adolescent Psychiatry,* April 2002: 378–85.

Sandler, Adrian D. "Attention-deficit/hyperactivity disorder and maternal smoking." *Journal of Developmental & Behavioral Pediatrics,* August 2002: 286.

"Smoking during pregnancy linked to ADHD in children." *Mental Health Weekly,* December 8, 2003: 8.

MEDICATION

Ahmann, Peter A., et al. "Placebo-controlled evaluation of amphetamine mixture—dextroamphetamine salts and amphetamine salts (Adderall): efficacy rate and side effects." *Pediatrics,* January 2001: 107.

Anderson, Carl M., et al. "Effects of methylphenidate on functional magnetic resonance relaxometry of the cerebellar vermis in boys with ADHD." *American Journal of Psychiatry,* August 2002: 1322–28.

Angold, Adrian; Alaattin Erkanli; Helen L. Egger; and E. Jane Costello. "Stimulant treatment for children: a community perspective." *Journal of American Academic Child Adolescent Psychiatry,* 2000: 975–94.

Bagwell, Catherine L.; Brooke S.G. Molina; William E. Pelham; and Betsy Hoza. "Attention-deficit/hyperactivity disorder and problems in peer relations: predictions from childhood to adolescence." *Journal of American Academic Child and Adolescent Psychiatry,* November 2001: 1285–92.

Bedard, Anne-Claude, et al. "Selective inhibition in children with attention-deficit/hyperactivity disorder off and on stimulant medication." *Journal of Abnormal Child Psychology,* June 2003: 315–27.

Biederman, Joseph; Frank A. Lopez; Samuel W. Boellner; and Mark C. Chandler. "A randomized, double-blind, placebo-controlled, parallel-group study of SLI381 (Adderall XR) in children with attention-deficit/hyperactivity disorder." *Pediatrics,* August 2002: 258–66.

Dosreis, Susan, et al. "Parental perceptions and satisfaction with stimulant medication for attention-deficit/hyperactivity disorder." *Journal of Developmental & Behavioral Pediatrics,* June 2003: 155–62.

Evans, Jeff. "ADHD medication may deter substance abuse, improve educational outcomes." *Clinical Psychiatry News,* February 2004: 55.

Farone, Stephen V. "A drug-placebo response curve analysis of the efficacy of a once-daily Oros[R] formulation of methylphenidate." *Journal of Developmental & Behavioral Pediatrics,* October 2002: 395.

Greenhill, Laurence L.; Robert L. Findling; and James M. Swanson. "A double-blind, placebo-controlled study of modified-release methylphenidate in children with attention-deficit/hyperactivity disorder." *Pediatrics,* March 2002: 512.

Guevara, J., et al. "Psychopharmacology. (psychotropic medication for attention-deficit/hyperactivity disorder)" *Journal of Developmental & Behavioral Pediatrics,* October 2002: 393–94.

Guevara, James, et al. "Psychotropic medication use in a population of children who have attention-deficit/hyperactivity disorder." *Pediatrics,* May 2002: 733–39.

Hazell, Philip L., and John E. Stuart. "A randomized controlled trial of clonidine added to psychostimulant medication for hyperactive and aggressive children." *Journal of the American Academy of Child and Adolescent Psychiatry,* August 2003: 886–94.

Hoagwood, Kimberly, et al. "Medication management of stimulants in pediatric practice settings: a national perspective." *Journal of Developmental and Behavioral Pediatrics,* 2000: 322–31.

James, Regina S., et al. "Double-blind, placebo-controlled study of single-dose amphetamine formulations in ADHD." *Journal of the American Academy of Child and Adolescent Psychiatry* November 2001: 1268–76.

Katusic, S. K., et al. "Psychopharmacologic treatment of ADHD in a population-based birth cohort: response to treatment and occurrence of side effects." *Journal of Developmental & Behavioral Pediatrics,* October 2002: 396.

Kratochvil, Christopher J., et al. "Atomoxetine and methyiphenidate treatment in children with ADHD: a prospective, randomized, open-label trial." *Journal of the American Academy of Child and Adolescent Psychiatry,* July 2002: 776–85.

Michelson, David, et al. "Once-daily atomoxetine treatment for children and adolescents with attention-deficit/hyperactivity disorder: a randomized, placebo-controlled study." *American Journal of Psychiatry,* November 2002: 1896–1901.

Miller, Karl E. "Once-a-day medication for ADHD treatment." *American Family Physician,* September 1, 2003: 956–60.

Pekkanen, J. "Making sense of Ritalin." *Reader's Digest,* June 2000: 153–58.

Pelham, William E., et al. "Behavioral versus behavioral and pharmacological treatment in ADHD children attending a summer treatment program." *Journal of Abnormal Child Psychology,* December 2000: 507–12.

Safer, Daniel J.; Julie M. Zito; and Eric M. Fine. "Increased methylpheidate usage for attention-deficit disorder in the 1990s." *Pediatrics,* December 1996: 1084–88.

Sandler, Adrian D. "Once-a-day Concerta methylphenidate versus three-times-daily methylphenidate in laboratory and natural settings." *Journal of Developmental & Behavioral Pediatrics,* December 2001: 449.

Teplin, Stuart W.; Catherine L. Grus; Adrian D. Sandler; and Michael I. Reiff. "An open-label, dose-ranging study of atomoxetine in children with attention-deficit/hyperactivity disorder." *Journal of Developmental & Behavioral Pediatrics,* February 2002: 64.

Teplin, Stuart W.; Catherine L. Grus; Adrian D. Sandler; and Michael I. Reiff. "Stimulant treatment for children: a community perspective." *Journal of Developmental & Behavioral Pediatrics,* December 2000: 454–59.

Teplin, Stuart W.; Catherine L. Grus; Adrian D. Sandler; and Michael I. Reiff. "Effects of stimulant medication treatment on mothers' and children's attributions for the behavior of children with attention-deficit/hyperactivity disorder." *Journal of Developmental & Behavioral Pediatrics,* December 2000: 454–59.

Tucha, Oliver, and Klaus W. Lange. "Effects of methylphenidate on kinematic aspects of handwriting in hyperactive boys." *Journal of Abnormal Child Psychology,* August 2001: 351–54.

Volkow, N. D., et al. "Is methylphenidate like cocaine? Studies on their pharmacokinetics and distribution in human brain." *Archives of General Psychiatry,* 1995: 456–63.

Wilens, Timothy E. *Straight Talk About Psychiatric Medications for Kids.* New York: Guilford Publications, 1998.

Wilens, Timothy, et al. "ADHD treatment with once-daily OROS methylphenidate: interim 12–month results from a long-team open-label study." *Journal of the American Academy of Child and Adolescent Psychiatry,* April 2003: 424–35.

OBSESSIVE-COMPULSIVE DISORDER AND AD/HD

Geller, Daniel A., et al. "Attention-deficit/hyperactivity disorder in children and adolescents with obsessive-compulsive disorder: Fact or artifact?" *Journal of the American Academy of Child and Adolescent Psychiatry,* January 2002: 52–58.

OPPOSITIONAL DEFIANT DISORDER AND AD/HD

Burns, G. Leonard, and James A. Walsh. "The influence of ADHD-hyperactivity/impulsivity symptoms on the development of oppositional defiant disorder symptoms in a 2–year longitudinal study." *Journal of Abnormal Child Psychology,* June 2002: 245–56.

Burns, G. Leonard, et al. "A confirmatory factor analysis on the DSM-IV ADHD and ODD symptoms: what is the best model for the organization of these symptoms?" *Journal of Abnormal Child Psychology,* 2001: 339–49.

Clark, Cheryl; Margot Prior; and Glynda J. Kinsella. "Do executive function deficits differentiate between adolescents with ADHD and oppositional defiant/conduct disorder? A neuropsychological study using the Six Elements Test and Hayling Sentence Completion Test." *Journal of Abnormal Child Psychology,* October 2000: 403–7.

Molina, Brooke S.G.; Bradley H. Smith; and William E. Pelham. "Factor structure and criterion validity of secondary school teacher ratings of ADHD and ODD." *Journal of Abnormal Child Psychology,* 2001: 71–82.

PRESCHOOLERS AND AD/HD

Connor, Daniel F. "Preschool attention-deficit hyperactivity disorder: A review of prevalence, diagnosis, neurobiology, and stimulant treatment." *Journal of Developmental & Behavioral Pediatrics,* February 2002: 1–9.

Coyle, Joseph T. "Psychotropic drug use in very young children." *Journal of the American Medical Association,* 2000: 1059.

Diller, Lawrence H. "Lessons from three year olds (attention-deficit hyperactivity disorder)." *Journal of Developmental & Behavioral Pediatrics,* February 2002: 10–12.

DuPaul, George J.; Kara E. McGoey; Tanya L. Eckert; and John VanBrakle. "Preschool children with attention-deficit/hyperactivity disorder: impairments in behavioral, social, and school functioning." *Journal of the American Academy of Child and Adolescent Psychiatry,* May 2001: 508–15.

Fraser, Kathleen M. "Too young for attention-deficit disorder? Views from preschool." *Journal of Developmental and Behavioral Pediatrics,* February 2002: 46–50.

Gadow, Kenneth D.; Joyce Sprafkin; and Edith E. Nolan. "DSM-IV symptoms in community and clinic preschool children." *Journal of the American Academy of Child and Adolescent Psychiatry,* December 2001: 1383–92.

Ghuman, Jaswinder Kaur, et al. "Psychostimulants in preschool children with attention-deficit/hyperactivity disorder: Clinical evidence from a developmental disorders institution." *Journal of the American Academy of Child and Adolescent Psychiatry,* May 2001: 516–20.

Reiff, Michael I. "Psychostimulants in preschool children with attention-deficit/hyperactivity disorder: Clinical evidence from a developmental disorders institution." *Journal of Developmental & Behavioral Pediatrics,* October 2001: 338–39.

Sandler, Adrian D. "Attention-deficit/hyperactivity disorder in preschoolers: Psychiatric comorbidity." *Journal of Developmental & Behavioral Pediatrics,* August 2002: 287–88.

Sonuga-Barke, Edmund J.S., et al. "Parent-based therapies for preschool attention-deficit/hyperactivity disorder: A randomized, controlled trial with a community sample." *Journal of the American Academy of Child and Adolescent Psychiatry,* April 2001: 402–5.

Zito, Julie Magno, et al. "Trends in the prescribing of psychotropic medications to preschoolers." *Journal of the American Medical Association,* February 23, 2000: 1025–32.

PRETERM BABIES

Bhutto, Adnan T., et al. "Cognitive and behavioral outcomes of school-aged children who were born preterm: A meta-analysis." *Journal of the American Medical Association,* August 14, 2002: 728–37.

Mick, Eric, et al. "Impact of low birth weight on attention-deficit/hyperactivity disorder." *Journal of Developmental & Behavioral Pediatrics,* February 2002: 16–22.

SEIZURES

Macias, Michelle M. "ADHD in children with seizure disorders: epidemiologic factors." *Journal of Developmental & Behavioral Pediatrics,* June 2003: 210.

Williams, Jane, et al. "Differentiating between seizures and attention-deficit/hyperactivity disorder (ADHD) in a pediatric population." *Clinical Pediatrics,* October 2002: 565–68.

Williams, Jane; Eldon G. Schulz; and May L. Griebel. "Seizure occurrence in children diagnosed with ADHD." *Clinical Pediatrics,* April 2001: 221–24.

SENSORY ISSUES

Belle Curve Records Inc. 888-357-5867 or www.bellecurve.com

Greene, Ross W. *The Explosive Child.* New York: First Quill Publishers, 2001.

Kranowitz, Carol Stock. *The Out-of-Sync Child*. New York: Perigee Trade, 1998. www.out-of-sync-child.com

Picker, Lauren. "When Children Feel Too Much—or Too Little." *Child*, December-January 2004: 62–68.

Sensory Integration International (www.sinetwork.org). www.sensorycomfort.com

SLEEP DISORDERS

Chervin, Ronald D., et al. "Inattention, hyperactivity, and symptoms of sleep-disordered breathing." *Pediatrics*, March 2002: 449–56.

O'Brien, Louise M., et al. "Sleep and neurobehavioral characteristics of 5- to 7-year-old children with parentally reported symptoms of attention-deficit/hyperactivity disorder." *Pediatrics*, March 2003: 554–63.

Owens, Judith A. "Parental and self-report of sleep in children with attention-deficit/hyperactivity disorder." *The Journal of the American Medical Association*, September 13, 2000: 1223–32.

Sandler, Adrian D. "Attention-deficit/hyperactivity disorder and sleep-disordered breathing." *Journal of Developmental & Behavioral Pediatrics*, August 2002: 287.

"Sleep disturbances high in ADHD children. (What's New in Research)" *The Brown University Child and Adolescent Behavior Letter*, February 2004: 4–5.

Stein, Daniel, et al. "Sleep disturbances in adolescents with symptoms of attention-deficit/hyperactivity disorder." *Journal of Learning Disabilities*, May–June 2002: 268–75.

SUBSTANCE ABUSE

Barkley, Russell A.; Mariellen Fischer; Lori Smallish; and Kenneth Fletcher. "Does the treatment of attention-deficit/hyperactivity disorder with stimulants contribute to drug use/abuse? A 13-year prospective study." *Pediatrics*, January 2003: 97–109.

McNamara, Damian. "Preliminary findings: uncontrolled ADHD associated with substance use in study." *Clinical Psychiatry News*, December 2003: 32.

Molina, Brooke S.G., and William E. Pelham, Jr. "Childhood predictors of adolescent substance use in a longitudinal study of children with ADHD." *Journal of Abnormal Psychology*, August 2003: 497–507.

Wagner, Karen Dineen. "Childhood ADHD and adolescent substance use." *Psychiatric Times*, April 1, 2004: 92.

Wellberry, Caroline. "Stimulants for ADHD do not cause substance abuse." *American Family Physician*, April 15, 2003: 1797–1804.

Wilens, Timothy E.; Stephen V. Faraone; Joseph Biederman; and Samantha Gunawardene. "Does stimulant therapy of attention-deficit/hyperactivity disorder beget later substance abuse? A meta-analytic review of the literature." *Pediatrics*, January 2003: 179–85.

TEENS AND AD/HD

Barkley, Russell A.; Kevin Murphy; and Denise Kwasnick. "Motor vehicle driving competencies and risk in teens and young adults with attention-deficit/hyperactivity disorder." *Pediatrics,* December 1996: 1089–95.

Barkley, Russell A.; Mariellen Fischer; Lori Smallish; and Kenneth Fletcher. "The persistence of attention-deficit/hyperactivity disorder into young adulthood as a function of reporting source and definition of disorder." *Journal of Abnormal Psychology,* 2002: 279–89.

"Better driving by teens with ADHD may be due Concerta." *Drug Week,* April 2, 2004: 34.

Fischer, Mariellen Fischer; Russell A. Barkley; Lori Smallish; and Kenneth Fletcher. "Young adult follow-up of hyperactive children: self-reported psychiatric disorders, comorbidity, and the role of childhood conduct problems and teen CD." *Journal of Abnormal Child Psychology,* October 2002: 463–75.

Minskoff, Esther H., and David Allsopp. *Academic Success Strategies for Adolescents with Learning Disabilities and ADHD.* Baltimore: Paul H. Brookes Publisher, 2002.

Woodward, L.; D. Fergusson; and L. J. Horwood. "Driving outcomes of young people with attentional difficulties in adolescence." *Journal of Developmental & Behavioral Pediatrics,* October 2000: 378–82.

TIC BEHAVIOR AND TOURETTE'S SYNDROME

Deputy, Stephen R. "Treatment of ADHD in children with tics: a randomized controlled trial." *Clinical Pediatrics,* November–December 2002: 736.

Gadow, Kenneth D.; Edith E. Nolan; Joyce Sprafkin; and Joseph Schwartz. "Tics and psychiatric comorbidity in children and adolescents." *Journal of the American Academy of Child and Adolescent Psychiatry,* January 2003: 29.

Mostofsky, Stewart H., et al. "Oculomotor abnormalities in boys with Tourette syndrome with and without ADHD." *Journal of the American Academy of Child and Adolescent Psychiatry,* December 2001: 1464–72.

Peterson, Bradley S.; Daniel S. Pine; Patricia Cohen; and Judith S. Brook. "Prospective, longitudinal study of tic, obsessive-compulsive, and attention-deficit/hyperactivity disorders in an epidemiological sample." *Journal of the American Academy of Child and Adolescent Psychiatry,* June 2001: 685–90.

Reiff, Michael I. "Tourette syndrome and ADHD." *Journal of Developmental & Behavioral Pediatrics,* June 2003: 214.

Spencer, Thomas, et al. "A double-blind comparison of desipramine and placebo in children and adolescents with chronic tic disorder and comorbid attention-deficit/hyperactivity disorder." *Archives of General Psychiatry,* July 2002: 649–56.

Sukhodolsky, Denis G., et al. "Disruptive behavior in children with Tourette's syndrome: association with ADHD comorbidity, tic severity, and functional impairment." *Journal of the American Academy of Child and Adolescent Psychiatry,* January 2003: 98–105.

Van Houten, Ben. "Tourette syndrome may affect ADHD patients: Up to one-third of ADHD patients." *Pediatric News,* March 2004: 27.

Resources

BOOKS

Amen, Daniel G. *Healing ADD: The Breakthrough Program That Allows You to See and Heal the Six Types of Attention-Deficit Disorder.* New York: Berkley Publishing Group, 2002.

Barkley, Russell A. *Taking Charge of ADHD.* Revised edition. New York: Guilford Publications, 2000.

Carpenter, Phyllis. *Sparky's Excellent Misadventures: My A.D.D. Journal by Me (Sparky).* Washington, DC: Magination Press American Psychological Association, 1999.

Cimera, Robert Evert. *Making ADHD a Gift.* Boca Raton, FL: CRC Press, 2002.

Corman, Cliff L., and Esther Trevino. *Eukee, the Jumpy Jumpy Elephant.* Plantation, FL: Specialty Press, 1995.

Diagnostic and Statistical Manual of Mental Disorders (DSM-IV). Washington, DC: American Psychiatric Association, 1994.

Flick, Grad L. *ADD/ADHD Behavior-Change Resource Kit: Ready-to-Use Strategies & Activities for Helping Children with Attention-Deficit Disorder.* Hoboken, NJ: Jossey-Bass, 2000.

Galvin, Matthew R. *Otto Learns About His Medicine: A Story About Medication for Children with ADHD.* Washington, DC: American Psychological Association, 2001.

Gordon, Michael. *Jumpin' Johnny Get Back to Work!: A Child's Guide to ADHD/Hyperactivity.* DeWitt, NY: GSI Publications, 1991.

Hallowell, Edward M., M.D.; and John J. Ratey, M.D. *Driven to Distraction.* New York: Simon & Schuster, 1994.

Harman, P. L. *The CHADD Information and Resource Guide to AD/HD.* Landover, MD: CHADD, 2001.

Hartmann, Thom. *Thom Hartmann's Complete Guide to ADHD: Help for Your Family at Home, School and Work*. Grass Valley, CA: Underwood Books, 2000.

Isaac, George. *Bipolar Not ADHD: Unrecognized Epidemic of Manic Depressive Illness in Children*. Lincoln, NE: IUniverse, 2001.

Janover, Caroline. *Zipper, the Kid with ADHD*. Rockville, MD: Woodbine House, 1997.

Kennedy, Diane, and Rebecca Banks. *ADHD-Autism Connection: A Step Toward More Accurate Diagnoses and Effective Treatments*. Colorado Springs, CO: WaterBrook Press, 2002.

Kravets, Marybeth, and Imy F. Wax. *The K&W Guide to Colleges for Students with Learning Disabilities or Attention-Deficit Disorder*. New York: Random House Information Group, 2003.

Kutscher, Martin L. *ADHD Book: Living Right Now!* Baltimore: Greenleaf Book Group, 2003.

Lacy, Shirley. *Hyperactivity/ADHD: New Solutions*. Bloomington, IN: 1stBooks Library, 2002.

Levy, Florence, and David A. Hay. *Attention, Genes and ADHD*. London: Taylor & Francis, 2003.

Maxmen, Jerrold S., and Nicholas G. Ward. *Psychotropic Drugs Fast Facts*. New York: W.W. Norton & Company, 2002.

Mooney, Jonathan, and David Cole. *Learning Outside the Lines: Two Ivy League Students with Learning Disabilities and ADHD Give You the Tools for Academic Success and Educational Revolution*. New York: Simon & Schuster Adult Publishing Group, 2000.

Mordasini, Don. *Wild Child: How You Can Help Your Child with Attention-deficit Disorder (ADD) and Other Behavioral Disorders*. Binghamton, NY: Haworth Press, 2001.

Moss, Deborah M. *Shelley, the Hyperactive Turtle*. Rockville, MD: Woodbine House, 1990.

Nadeau, Kathleen. *Help4ADD@Highschool*. Bethesda, MD: Advantage Books, 1998.

Nylund, David. *Treating Huckleberry Finn: A New Narrative Approach to Working with Kids Diagnosed ADD/ADHD*. Hoboken, NJ: John Wiley & Sons, 2002.

Parker, Harvey C. *Problem Solver Guide for Students with ADHD*. Plantation, FL: Specialty Press, 2001.

Pliszka, Steven R.; Caryn L. Carlson; and James M. Swanson. *ADHD with Comorbid Disorders: Clinical Assessment and Management*. New York: Guilford Publications, 2001.

Power, Thomas J.; Dina F. Habboushe; and James L. Karustis. *Homework Success for Children with ADHD: A Family-School Intervention Program*. New York: Guilford Publications, 2001.

Quinn, Patricia O. *ADD and the College Student: A Guide for High School and College Students with Attention-Deficit Disorder*. Washington, DC: Magination Press/American Psychological Assocation, April 2001.

Reif, Sandra F., and Ariel Rief (illustrator). *The ADHD Book of Lists*. Hoboken, NJ: John Wiley & Sons, 2003.

Reiff, Michael I. *ADHD: A Complete and Authoritative Guide*. Elk Grove Village, IL: American Academy of Pediatrics, 2004.

Stein, David B. *Unraveling The Add/Adhd Fiasco*. Kansas City, MO: Andrews McMeel Publishing, 2001.

Swanberg, Dennis; Diane Passno; Kathy Davis; and Mick Silva. *Why A.D.H.D Doesn't Mean Disaster*. Wheaton, IL: Tyndale House Publishers, 2003.

Taylor, John F. *Helping Your ADD Child: Hundreds of Practical Solutions for Parents and Teachers of ADD Children and Teens (With or Without Hyperactivity).* Victoria, B.C., Canada: Crown Publishing Group, 2001.

Teaching Teens with ADD and ADHD: A Quick Reference Guide for Teachers and Parents. Bethesda, MD: Woodbine House, 2000.

Timmerman, John H. *Real Solutions for Living with ADHD.* Ann Arbor, MI: Servant Publications, 2002.

Weiss, Margaret; Gabrielle Weiss; and Lily Trockenberg Hechtman. *ADHD in Adulthood: A Guide to Current Theory, Diagnosis, and Treatment.* Baltimore: Johns Hopkins University Press, 2001.

Wender, Paul H. *ADHD: Attention-Deficit Hyperactivity Disorder in Children and Adults.* New York: Oxford University Press, 2001.

Wilens, Timothy E. *Straight Talk About Psychiatric Medications for Kids.* New York: Guilford Publications, 1998.

Zimmitt, Debbie. *Eddie Enough!* Rockville, MD: Woodbine House, 2001.

PERIODICAL ARTICLES

"ADHD often comorbid with affective illness. (What's New in Research)." *The Brown University Child and Adolescent Behavior Letter,* January 2004: 4–5.

"ADHD symptoms often treated only during school day." *Mental Health Weekly,* January 5, 2004: 8.

Abikoff, Howard. "Tailored Psychosocial Treatments for ADHD: The Search for a Good Fit." *Journal of Clinical Child Psychology,* March 2001: 122.

Ahmann, Peter A., et al. "Placebo-controlled evaluation of amphetamine mixture—dextro-amphetamine salts and amphetamine salts (Adderall): efficacy rate and side effects." *Pediatrics,* January 2001: 107.

American Academy of Pediatrics, Subcommittee on Attention-Deficit/Hyperactivity Disorder and Committee on Quality Improvement. "Clinical practice guideline: treatment of the school-aged child with attention-deficit/hyperactivity disorder." *Pediatrics,* 2001: 1033–44.

Anderson, Carl M., et al. "Effects of methylphenidate on functional magnetic resonance relaxometry of the cerebellar vermis in boys with ADHD." *American Journal of Psychiatry,* August 2002: 1322–28.

Arnold, L. Eugene, et al. "Nine months of multicomponent behavioral treatment for ADHD and effectiveness of MTA fading procedures." *Journal of Abnormal Child Psychology,* February 2004: 39–51.

Arons, Bernard S.; Judith Katz-Leavy; Alexandra C. Wittig; and E. Wayne Holden. "Too young for ADHD: the potential role of systems of care." *Journal of Developmental and Behavioral Pediatrics,* February 2002: S57–63.

Bagwell, Catherine L.; Brooke S.G. Molina; William E. Pelham; and Betsy Hoza. "Attention-deficit/hyperactivity disorder and problems in peer relations: predictions from childhood to adolescence." *Journal of American Academic Child and Adolescent Psychiatry,* November 2001: 1285–92.

Barbaresi, William J., et al. "How common is attention-deficit/hyperactivity disorder?

Incidence in a population-based birth cohort in Rochester, Minn." *Archives of Pediatrics & Adolescent Medicine,* March 2002: 217–24.

Barkley, Russell A. "Genetics of childhood disorders: XVII. ADHD, Part 1: The executive functions and ADHD." *Journal of the American Academy of Child and Adolescent Psychiatry,* August 2000: 1064–71.

Bauermeister, Jose J., et al. "Stimulant and psychosocial treatment of ADHD in Latino/ Hispanic children." *Journal of the American Academy of Child and Adolescent Psychiatry,* July 2003: 851–55.

Bedard, Anne-Claude; Rhonda Martinussen; Abel Ickowicz; and Rosemary Tannock. "Methylphenidate improves visual-spatial memory in children with attention-deficit/ hyperactivity disorder." *Journal of the American Academy of Child and Adolescent Psychiatry,* March 2004: 260–68.

Bedard, Anne-Claude Bedard, et al. "Selective inhibition in children with attention-deficit hyperactivity disorder off and on stimulant medication." *Journal of Abnormal Child Psychology,* June 2003: 315–27.

Biederman, Joseph. "Attention-deficit/hyperactivity disorder: a life span perspective." *Journal of Clinical Psychiatry,* 1998: 4–16.

Biederman, Joseph; Stephen V. Faraone; and Michael C. Monuteaux. "Differential effect of environmental adversity by gender: Rutter's index of adversity in a group of boys and girls with and without ADHD." *American Journal of Psychiatry,* September 2002: 1556–62.

Biederman, Joseph, et al. "Influence of gender on attention-deficit/hyperactivity disorder in children referred to a psychiatric clinic." *American Journal of Psychiatry,* January 2002: 36–42.

Biederman, Joseph, et al. "Growth deficits and attention-deficit/hyperactivity disorder revisited: Impact of gender, development, and treatment." *Pediatrics,* May 2003: 1010–16.

Biederman, Joseph; Frank A. Lopez; Samuel W. Boellner; and Mark C. Chandler. "A randomized, double-blind, placebo-controlled, parallel-group study of SLI381 (Adderall XR) in children with attention-deficit/hyperactivity disorder." *Pediatrics,* August 2002: 258–66.

Bhutto, Adnan T., et al. "Cognitive and behavioral outcomes of school-aged children who were born preterm: A meta-analysis." *The Journal of the American Medical Association,* August 14, 2002: 728–37.

Burns, G. Leonard, and James A. Walsh. "The influence of ADHD-hyperactivity/impulsivity symptoms on the development of oppositional defiant disorder symptoms in a 2-year longitudinal study." *Journal of Abnormal Child Psychology,* June 2002: 245–56.

Bussing, Regina, et al. "Social networks, caregiver strain, and utilization of mental health services among elementary school students at high risk for ADHD." *Journal of the American Academy of Child and Adolescent Psychiatry,* July 2003: 842–50.

Carlson, Caryn L.; Jane E. Booth; Misung Shin; and Will H. Canu. "Parent-, teacher-, and self-rated motivational styles in ADHD subtypes." *Journal of Learning Disabilities,* March–April 2002: 104–13.

"CHADD launches Online ADHD library." *The Brown University Child and Adolescent Behavior Letter,* April 2004: 2.

Chatfield, Joanne. "AAP Guideline on Treatment of Children with ADHD. (Committee on Quality Improvement and the Subcommittee on Attention-Deficit/Hyperactivity

Disorder of the American Academy of Pediatrics)." *American Family Physician,* February 15, 2002: 726.

Chi, Terry C., and Stephen P. Hinshaw. "Mother–child relationships of children with ADHD: the role of maternal depressive symptoms and depression-related distortions." *Journal of Abnormal Child Psychology,* August 2002: 387–400.

Chronis, A. M., et al. "Psychotropic drug treatments." *Journal of Developmental & Behavioral Pediatrics,* June 2003: 212–13.

Clark, Cheryl; Margot Prior; and Glynda Kinsella. "The relationship between executive function abilities, adaptive behaviour, and academic achievement in children with externalising behaviour problems." *Journal of Child Psychology and Psychiatry and Allied Disciplines,* September 2002: 785–96.

Combs, Jerome T. "Lack of right ear advantage in patients with attention-deficit/hyperactivity disorder." *Clinical Pediatrics,* May 2002: 231–34.

"Comorbidities cost ADHD patients." *Clinical Psychiatry News,* January 2004: 34.

Connor, Daniel F. "Preschool attention-deficit/hyperactivity disorder: a review of prevalence, diagnosis, neurobiology, and stimulant treatment." *Journal of Developmental & Behavioral Pediatrics,* February 2002: 1–9.

Connor, Daniel F., et al. "Correlates of comorbid psychopathology in children with ADHD." *Journal of the American Academy of Child and Adolescent Psychiatry,* February 2003: 193–200.

Connor, Daniel F., et al. "Psychopharmacology and aggression; I: A meta-analysis of stimulant effects on overt/covert aggression–related behaviors in ADHD." *Journal of the American Academy of Child and Adolescent Psychiatry,* March 2002: 253–61.

Cox, Daniel J., et al. "Impact of methylphenidate delivery profiles on driving performance of adolescents with attention-deficit/hyperactivity disorder: a pilot study." *Journal of the American Academy of Child and Adolescent Psychiatry,* March 2004: 269–75.

Cox, Emily R.; Brenda R. Motheral; Rochelle R. Henderson; and Doug Mager. "Geographic variation in the prevalence of stimulant medication use among children 5 to 14 years old: Results from a commercially insured US sample." *Pediatrics,* February 2003: 237–43.

Crone, Eveline A.; J. Richard Jennings; and Maurits W. van der Molen. "Sensitivity to interference and response contingencies in attention-deficit/hyperactivity disorder." *Journal of Child Psychology and Psychiatry and Allied Disciplines,* February 2003: 214–26.

Cunningham, Charles E., and Michael H. Boyle. "Preschoolers at risk for attention-deficit/hyperactivity disorder and oppositional defiant disorder: family, parenting, and behavioral correlates." *Journal of Abnormal Child Psychology,* December 2002: 555–69.

Cutting, Laurie E.; Christine W. Koth; E. Mark Mahone; and Martha B. Denckla. "Evidence for unexpected weaknesses in learning in children with attention-deficit/hyperactivity disorder without reading disabilities." *Journal of Learning Disabilities,* May–June 2003: 259–69.

Deputy, Stephen R. "Epileptiform abnormalities in children with attention-deficit/hyperactivity disorder." *Clinical Pediatrics,* November–December 2002: 737.

DeVeaugh-Geiss, Joseph, et al. "GW320659 for the treatment of attention-deficit/hyperactivity disorder in children." *Journal of the American Academy of Child and Adolescent Psychiatry,* August 2002: 914–20.

Dosreis, Susan, et al. "Parental perceptions and satisfaction with stimulant medication for attention-deficit/hyperactivity disorder." *Journal of Developmental & Behavioral Pediatrics,* June 2003: 155–62.

Durston, Sarah, et al. "Magnetic resonance imaging of boys with attention-deficit/hyperactivity disorder and their unaffected siblings." *Journal of the American Academy of Child and Adolescent Psychiatry,* March 2004: 332–40.

El-Sayed, Eman; Jan-Olov Larsson; Hans E. Persson; and Per-Anders Rydelius. "Altered cortical activity in children with attention-deficit/hyperactivity disorder during attentional load task." *Journal of the American Academy of Child and Adolescent Psychiatry,* July 2002: 811–19.

Ernst, Monique, et al. "Neural substrates of decision making in adults with attention-deficit/hyperactivity disorder." *American Journal of Psychiatry,* June 2003: 1061–70.

Evans, Jeff. "ADHD medication may deter substance abuse, improve educational outcomes." *Clinical Psychiatry News,* February 2004: 55.

Evans, Jeff. "ADHD Rx can lessen social risks: Substance abuse, school issues." *Pediatric News,* February 2004: 25.

"Experts clarify guidelines for ADHD and disruptive behavior disorders (International Consensus Statement)." *The Brown University Child and Adolescent Behavior Letter,* February 2004: 1–3.

Faraone, Stephen V. "A drug-placebo response curve analysis of the efficacy of a once-daily Oros[R] formulation of methylphenidate." *Journal of Developmental & Behavioral Pediatrics,* October 2002: 395.

Faraone, Stephen V., et al. "Does parental ADHD bias maternal reports of ADHD sym toms in children?" *Journal of Consulting and Clinical Psychology,* February 2003: 168–75.

"FOCUS study examines differences between Concerta, Strattera for ADHD symptoms." *The Brown University Child and Adolescent Psychopharmacology Update,* February 2004: 3.

Fraser, Kathleen M. "Too young for attention deficit disorder? Views from preschool." *Journal of Developmental and Behavioral Pediatrics,* February 2002: 46–50.

Geller, Daniel A., et al. "Attention-deficit/hyperactivity disorder in children and adolescents with obsessive-compulsive disorder: fact or artifact?" *Journal of the American Academy of Child and Adolescent Psychiatry,* January 2002: 52–58.

"Gender and familial associations are linked to ADHD and major depression." *Mental Health Weekly Digest,* January 18, 2004: 9.

Gephart, Harlan R. "One hundred years of managing ADHD—and where are we?" *Contemporary Pediatrics,* December 2003: 10.

Gillberg, Christopher, and Linda De Souza. "Head circumference in autism, asperger syndrome, and ADHD: a comparative study." *Journal of the American Academy of Child and Adolescent Psychiatry,* January 2003: 115.

Glascoe, Frances Page. "Safety words inventory and literacy screener: standardization and validation (attention-deficit with hyperactivity disorder diagnosis)." *Clinical Pediatrics,* November–December 2002: 697–704.

Gorskie, Peter A. "Racing Cain." *Journal of Developmental and Behavioral Pediatrics,* April 2002: 95.

Greenhill, Laurence L.; Robert L. Findling; and James M. Swanson. "A double-blind, placebo-controlled study of modified-release methylphenidate in children with attention-deficit/hyperactivity disorder." *Pediatrics,* March 2002: 512.

Gregg, Noel; Chris Coleman; Robert B. Stennett; and Mark Davis. "Discourse complexity of college writers with and without disabilities: a multidimensional analysis." *Journal of Learning Disabilities,* January–February 2002: 23–38.

Grus, Catherine L. "Attention-deficit/hyperactivity disorder and neuropsychological profiles." *Journal of Developmental & Behavioral Pediatrics,* April 2002: 120.

Grus, Catherine L. "Attention-deficit/hyperactivity disorder: social skills training." *Journal of Developmental & Behavioral Pediatrics,* August 2003: 295.

Grus, Catherine L.; Adrian D. Sandler; and Michael I. Reiff. "Attention-deficit/hyperactivity disorder." *Journal of Developmental & Behavioral Pediatrics,* June 2002: 186–87.

Guevara, J., et al. "Psychopharmacology (psychotropic medication for attention-deficit/hyperactivity disorder)." *Journal of Developmental & Behavioral Pediatrics,* October 2002: 393–94.

Guevara, James, et al. "Psychotropic medication use in a population of children who have attention-deficit/hyperactivity disorder." *Pediatrics,* May 2002: 733–39.

Harel, Ephat H., and William D. Brown. "Attention-deficit hyperactivity disorder in elementary school children in Rhode Island: associated psychosocial factors and medications used." *Clinical Pediatrics,* July–August 2003: 497–503.

Harpin, V.; S. Prasad; S. Zhang; and D. Michelson. "Atomoxetine in the long-term prevention of relapse in ADHD." *Archives of Disease in Childhood,* April 2004: A2–3.

Hazell, Philip L.; Vaughan Carr; Terry J. Lewin; and Ketrina Sly. "Manic symptoms in young males with ADHD predict functioning but not diagnosis after 6 years." *Journal of the American Academy of Child and Adolescent Psychiatry,* May 2003: 552–61.

Hazell, Philip L., and John E. Stuart. "A randomized controlled trial of clonidine added to psychostimulant medication for hyperactive and aggressive children." *Journal of the American Academy of Child and Adolescent Psychiatry,* August 2003: 886–94.

Heiligenstein, Eric; Liza M. Conyers; Andrew R. Berns; and Michelle A. Smith. "Preliminary Normative Data on DSM-IV Attention-Deficit/Hyperactivity Disorder in College Students." *Journal of Abnormal Psychology,* November 2002: 659–64.

Hill, Jonathan. "Biological, psychological and social processes in the conduct disorders." *Journal of Child Psychology and Psychiatry and Allied Disciplines,* January 2002: 133.

Hinshaw, Stephen P. "Moderators and mediators of treatment response for children with attention-deficit/hyperactivity disorder: the multimodal treatment study of children with attention-deficit/hyperactivity disorder." *Journal of the American Medical Association,* March 22, 2000: 1550–51.

Hoheb, Marisa. "Brain burn: millions of kids have attention-deficit/hyperactivity disorder (ADHD): Meet one of them and find out how she copes with this difficult ailment." *Scholastic Choices,* February–March 2004: 11–15.

Kalff, Ariane C., et al. "Neurocognitive performance of 5- and 6-year-old children who met criteria for attention-deficit/hyperactivity disorder at 18 months follow-up." *Journal of Abnormal Child Psychology,* December 2002: 589–98.

Katusic, S. K., et al. "Psychopharmacologic treatment of ADHD in a population-based birth cohort: response to treatment and occurrence of side effects." *Journal of Developmental & Behavioral Pediatrics,* October 2002: 396.

Khilnani, Sonya; Tiffany Field; Maria Hernandez-Reif; and Saul Schanberg. "Massage therapy improves mood and behavior of students with attention-deficit/hyperactivity disorder." *Adolescence,* Winter 2003: 623–38.

Konrad, Kerstin; Thomas Gunther; Charlotte Hanisch; and Beate Herpertz-Dahlmann. "Differential effects of methylphenidate on attentional functions in children with attention-deficit/hyperactivity disorder." *Journal of the American Academy of Child and Adolescent Psychiatry,* February 2004: 191–98.

Kratochvil, Christopher J., et al. "Atomoxetine and methyiphenidate treatment in children with ADHD: a prospective, randomized, open-label trial." *Journal of the American Academy of Child and Adolescent Psychiatry,* July 2002: 776–85.

Kube, David A.; Mario C. Petersen; and Frederick B. Palmer. "Attention-deficit/hyperactivity disorder: comorbidity and medication use." *Clinical Pediatrics,* September 2002: 461–70.

Kutcher, S., et al. "Experts clarify guidelines for ADHD and disruptive behavior disorders. (International Consensus Statement)." *Brown University Child and Adolescent Psychopharmacology Update,* February 2004: 1–4.

Lawrence, Vivienne, et al. "ADHD outside the laboratory: boys' executive function performance on tasks in videogame play and on a visit to the zoo." *Journal of Abnormal Child Psychology,* October 2002: 447–62.

Lesesne, Catherine A.; Susanna N. Visser; and Carla P. White. "Attention-deficit/hyperactivity disorder in school-aged children: association with maternal mental health and use of health care resources." *Pediatrics,* May 2003: 1232–37.

Leslie, L. K.; J. Weckerly; R.E.G. Pearson; and A. McDaniel. "Implementing AAP (American Academy of Pediatrics) guidelines for ADHD diagnosis in pediatric offices." *Journal of Developmental & Behavioral Pediatrics,* October 2002: 396–97.

Levy, Florence. "Project for a scientific psychiatry in the 21st century." *Journal of the American Academy of Child and Adolescent Psychiatry,* April 2003: 385.

Lorch, Elizabeth Pugzles, et al. "Difficulties in comprehending causal relations among children with ADHD: the role of cognitive engagement." *Journal of Abnormal Psychology,* February 2004: 56–63.

Macias, Michelle M. "ADHD and stimulant treatment: risk for adult drug abuse." *Journal of Developmental & Behavioral Pediatrics,* June 2003: 209–10.

"Managing ADHD: the full-time disorder." *Medical Economics,* March 19, 2004: 6–8.

Mattison, Richard E., et al. "A DSM-IV–referenced teacher rating scale for use in clinical management." *Journal of the American Academy of Child and Adolescent Psychiatry,* April 2003: 442–49.

Max, Jeffrey E., et al. "Putamen lesions and the development of attention-deficit/hyperactivity symptomatology." *Journal of the American Academy of Child and Adolescent Psychiatry,* May 2002: 563–71.

McCracken, James T., et al. "Analog classroom assessment of a once-daily mixed amphetamine formulation, SLI381 (Adderall XR), in children with ADHD." *Journal of the American Academy of Child and Adolescent Psychiatry,* June 2003: 673–83.

McGee, Rob, et al. "The long-term significance of teacher-rated hyperactivity and reading ability in childhood: findings from two longitudinal studies." *Journal of Child Psychology and Psychiatry and Allied Disciplines,* November 2002: 1004–1017.

McGough, James J., et al. "Pharmacokinetics of SLI381 (Adderall XR), an extended-release formulation of Adderall." *Journal of the American Academy of Child and Adolescent Psychiatry,* June 2003: 684–92.

McInnes, Alison; Tom Humphries; Sheilah Hogg-Johnson; and Rosemary Tannock. "Listening comprehension and working memory are impaired in attention-deficit/hyperactivity disorder irrespective of language impairment." *Journal of Abnormal Child Psychology,* August 2003: 427–43.

McNamara, Damian. "ADHD medication does not alter height or weight." *Clinical Psychiatry News,* February 2004: 55.

McNamara, Damian. "Atomoxetine for ADHD doesn't worsen tics: Nonstimulant alternative." *Pediatric News,* January 2004: 22.

McNamara, Damian. "Extended-release ADHD drugs beat placebo." *Clinical Psychiatry News,* February 2004: 55.

McNamara, Damian. "Stimulants for ADHD don't alter height or weight: 5–year follow-up study." *Pediatric News,* February 2004: 23.

Mehta, Satwant Kaur, and Joseph P. Horrigan. "Oral flower essences for ADHD." *Journal of the American Academy of Child and Adolescent Psychiatry,* August 2002: 895–96.

Michelson, David, et al. "Once-daily atomoxetine treatment for children and adolescents with attention-deficit/hyperactivity disorder: A randomized, placebo-controlled study." *American Journal of Psychiatry,* November 2002: 1896–1901.

Mick, Eric, et al. "Impact of low birth weight on attention-deficit/hyperactivity disorder." *Journal of Developmental & Behavioral Pediatrics,* February 2002: 16–22.

Miller, Karl E. "Once-a-day medication for ADHD treatment." *American Family Physician,* September 1, 2003: 956–60.

Miranda, Ana; Maria Jesus Presentacion; and Manuel Sorian. "Effectiveness of a school-based multicomponent program for the treatment of children with ADHD." *Journal of Learning Disabilities,* November–December 2002: 546–62.

Morantz, Carrie, and Brian Torrey. "Guidelines on diagnosis and management of ADHD." *American Family Physician,* September 1, 2003: 971–74.

Nattrass, K., et al. "In puppy love: How an assistance dog can enhance the life of a child with a disability." *Contemporary Pediatrics,* January 2004: 57–60.

"New look at ADHD data suggests lasting effect of behavioral treatment (The NIMH Multimodal Treatment Study)." *The Brown University Child and Adolescent Behavior Letter,* February 2004: 7.

Nigg, Joel T.; Lisa G. Blaskey; Cynthia L. Huang-Pollock; and Marsha D. Rappley. "Neuropsychological executive functions and DSM-IV ADHD subtypes." *Journal of the American Academy of Child and Adolescent Psychiatry,* January 2002: 59–66.

Olfson, Mark; Marc J. Gameroff; Steven C. Marcus; and Peter S. Jensen. "National trends in the treatment of attention-deficit/hyperactivity disorder." *American Journal of Psychiatry,* June 2003: 1071–76.

Owens, Elizabeth B., et al. "Which treatment for whom for ADHD? Moderators of treatment response in the MTA." *Journal of Consulting and Clinical Psychology,* June 2003: 540–52.

Pearson, Deborah A., et al. "Treatment effects of methylphenidate on behavioral adjustment in children with mental retardation and ADHD." *Journal of the American Academy of Child and Adolescent Psychiatry,* February 2003: 209–16.

Pentikis, Helen S.; Roy D. Simmons; Michael F. Benedict; and Simon J. Hatch. "Methyl-phenidate bioavailability in adults when an extended-release multiparticulate formulation is administered sprinkled on food or as an intact capsule." *Journal of the American Academy of Child and Adolescent Psychiatry,* April 2002: 443–49.

Pirisi, Angela. "ADHD may predict later substance use problems." *The Journal of Addiction and Mental Health,* Winter 2003: 6–7.

Pliszka, Steven R., et al. "A feasibility study of the Children's Medication Algorithm Project (CMAP) Algorithm for the Treatment of ADHD." *Journal of the American Academy of Child and Adolescent Psychiatry,* March 2003: 279–87.

Power, Thomas J.; Tracy E. Costigan; Ricardo B. Eiraldi; and Stephen S. Leff. "Variations in anxiety and depression as a function of ADHD subtypes defined by DSM-IV: Do subtype differences exist or not?" *Journal of Abnormal Child Psychology,* February 2004: 27–37.

Quallich, Susanne A. "Linking ADHD and voiding dysfunction." *Urologic Nursing,* February 2004: 55.

Rappley, Marsha D., et al. "Patterns of psychotropic medication use in very young children with attention-deficit/hyperactivity disorder." *Journal of Developmental & Behavioral Pediatrics,* February 2002: 23–30.

Rasmussen, Erik R., et al. "Replication of the latent class structure of attention-deficit/hyperactivity disorder (ADHD) subtypes in a sample of Australian twins." *Journal of Child Psychology and Psychiatry and Allied Disciplines,* November 2002: 1018–28.

Reid, Robert; Paul Hakendorf; and Brenton Prosser. "Use of psychostimulant medication for ADHD in South Australia." *Journal of the American Academy of Child and Adolescent Psychiatry,* August 2002: 906–13.

Reiff, Michael I. "Attention-deficit/hyperactivity disorder: Quality of life measurement." *Journal of Developmental & Behavioral Pediatrics,* October 2002: 391.

Reiff, Michael I., and Adrian D. Sandler. "ADHD and pharmacotherapy." *Journal of Developmental & Behavioral Pediatrics,* April 2002: 120–21.

Renz, Kelly, et al. "On-line story representation in boys with attention-deficit/hyperactivity disorder." *Journal of Abnormal Child Psychology,* February 2003: 93–104.

Rieppi, Ricardo, et al. "Socioeconomic status as a moderator of ADHD treatment outcomes." *Journal of the American Academy of Child and Adolescent Psychiatry,* March 2002: 269–77.

Rowland, Andrew S., et al. "Prevalence of medication treatment for attention-deficit/hyperactivity disorder among elementary school children in Johnston County, North Carolina." *The American Journal of Public Health,* February 2002: 231–34.

Rubia, Katya, et al. "Motor timing deficits in community and clinical boys with hyperactive behavior: the effect of methylphenidate on motor timing." *Journal of Abnormal Child Psychology,* June 2003: 301–13.

Rubin, K. H.; K. B. Burgess; K. M. Dwyer; and P. D. Hastings. "Temperament." *Journal of Developmental & Behavioral Pediatrics,* June 2003: 213–14.

Rucklidge, Julia J., and Rosemary Tannock. "Neuropsychological profiles of adolescents with ADHD: effects of reading difficulties and gender." *Journal of Child Psychology and Psychiatry and Allied Disciplines,* November 2002: 988–1003.

Sadovsky, Richard. "The management of Attention-Deficit/Hyperactivity Disorder." *American Family Physician,* March 1, 2002: 931–35.

Sandler, Adrian D. "Attention-deficit/hyperactivity disorder prevalence." *Journal of Developmental & Behavioral Pediatrics,* August 2002: 287.

Sandler, Adrian D. "Attention-deficit/hyperactivity disorder practice parameter." *Journal of Developmental & Behavioral Pediatrics,* August 2002: 286–87.

Sandler, Adrian D. "Attention-deficit/hyperactivity disorder and docosahexaenoic acid supplementation." *Journal of Developmental & Behavioral Pediatrics,* August 2002: 286.

Sandler, Adrian D. "Psychopharmacology." *Journal of Developmental & Behavioral Pediatrics,* February 2003: 82–83.

Scheres, Anouk, et al. "The effect of methylphenidate on three forms of response inhibition in boys with AD/HD." *Journal of Abnormal Child Psychology,* February 2003: 105–20.

Sharp, Wendy S., et al. "Monozygotic twins discordant for attention-deficit/hyperactivity disorder: ascertainment and clinical characteristics." *Journal of the American Academy of Child and Adolescent Psychiatry,* January 2003: 93–97.

Sonuga-Barke, Edmund J. S.; David Daley; and Margaret Thompson. "Does maternal ADHD reduce the effectiveness of parent training for preschool children's ADHD?" *Journal of the American Academy of Child and Adolescent Psychiatry,* June 2002: 696–702.

Sonuga-Barke, Edmund J. S. "Interval length and time-use by children with AD/HD: A comparison of four models." *Journal of Abnormal Child Psychology,* June 2002: 257–64.

Sprafkin, Joyce, et al. "A DSM-IV-referenced screening instrument for preschool children: The Early Childhood Inventory-4." *Journal of the American Academy of Child and Adolescent Psychiatry,* May 2002: 604–12.

Stroes, Ad; Ed Alberts; and Jaap J. VanDer Meere. "Boys with ADHD in social interaction with a nonfamiliar adult: an observational study." *Journal of the American Academy of Child and Adolescent Psychiatry,* March 2003: 295–302.

"Study: Treatment of ADHD should also include parents." *Mental Health Weekly,* January 12, 2004: 4.

"Study links ADHD drugs to growth delays, though permanent effects not known." *Drug Week,* April 30, 2004: 30.

Sullivan, Michele G. "ADHD may be behind many mental health issues: Undertreated, misdiagnosed." *Family Practice News,* February 15, 2004: 21.

Sullivan, Michele G. "Undertreated, misdiagnosed: Adult ADHD needs attention from physicians." *Internal Medicine News,* March 1, 2004: 48.

Sullivan, Michele G. "Undiagnosed ADHD affects millions of adults." *Clinical Psychiatry News,* February 2004: 4.

Swanson, James M., et al. "A comparison of once-daily extended-release methylphenidate formulations in children with attention-deficit/hyperactivity disorder in the laboratory school (The Comacs Study)." *Pediatrics,* March 2004: 612–13.

Swanson, James M., et al. "Efficacy of a new pattern of delivery of methylphenidate for the treatment of ADHD: effects on activity level in the classroom and on the playground." *Journal of the American Academy of Child and Adolescent Psychiatry,* November 2002: 1306–14.

Swanson, James M., et al. "Response to commentary on the Multimodal Treatment Study of ADHD (MTA): mining the meaning of the MTA." *Journal of Abnormal Child Psychology,* August 2002: 327–32.

Teplin, Stuart W.; Catherine L. Grus; Adrian D. Sandler; and Michael I. Reiff. "An open-label, dose-ranging study of atomoxetine in children with attention-deficit/hyperactivity disorder." *Journal of Developmental & Behavioral Pediatrics,* February 2002: 64.

Teplin, Stuart W.; Catherine L. Grus; Andrian D. Sandler; and Michael I. Reiff. "Psychophysiological responses in ADHD boys with and without conduct disorder: implications for adult antisocial behavior." *Journal of Developmental & Behavioral Pediatrics,* February 2002: 61.

Tercyak, Kenneth P.; Caryn Lerman; and Janet Audrain. "Association of attention-deficit/hyperactivity disorder symptoms with levels of cigarette smoking in a community sample of adolescents." *Journal of the American Academy of Child and Adolescent Psychiatry,* July 2002: 799–805.

Todd, Richard D., et al. "Discrimination of DSM-IV and latent class attention-deficit/hyperactivity disorder subtypes by educational and cognitive performance in a population-based sample of child and adolescent twins." *Journal of the American Academy of Child and Adolescent Psychiatry,* July 2002: 820–28.

Tutty, Steve; Harlan Gephart; and Kathie Wurzbacher. "Enhancing behavioral and social skill functioning in children newly diagnosed with attention-deficit/hyperactivity disorder in a pediatric setting." *Journal of Developmental & Behavioral Pediatrics,* February 2003: 51–57.

Upadhyaya, Himanshu P.; Kathleen T. Brady; and Wei Wang. "Bupropion SR in adolescents with comorbid ADHD and nicotine dependence: a pilot study." *Journal of the American Academy of Child and Adolescent Psychiatry,* February 2004: 199–205.

Van Dyck, Christopher H., et al. "Unaltered dopamine transporter availability in adult attention-deficit/hyperactivity disorder." *American Journal of Psychiatry,* February 2002: 309–11.

Vastag, Brian. "More children on CNS drugs." *The Journal of the American Medical Association,* April 17, 2002: 1930.

Vreugdenhil, Coby, et al. "Psychiatric disorders in a representative sample of incarcerated boys in the Netherlands." *Journal of the American Academy of Child and Adolescent Psychiatry,* January 2004: 97–104.

Weesing, V. Robin, and John R. Weisz. "Mechanisms of action in youth psychotherapy." *Journal of Child Psychology and Psychiatry and Allied Disciplines,* January 2002: 3–28.

Wender, Esther. "ADHD symptoms and parent-teacher agreement." *Journal of Developmental & Behavioral Pediatrics.*

Wender, Esther H. "Attention-deficit/hyperactivity disorder: Is it common? Is it overtreated?" *Archives of Pediatrics & Adolescent Medicine,* March 2002: 209–10.

Westlake, Laurie. "Disorderly conduct: It took years to discover the source of my son's behavior problems—ADHD." *Today's Christian Woman,* March–April 2004: 24–27.

Weyandt, Lisa L.; Linda Mitzlaff; and Laura Thomas. "The relationship between intelligence and performance on the Test of Variables of Attention (TOVA)." *Journal of Learning Disabilities,* March–April 2002: 114–20.

Weyandt, Lisa L., et al. "The Internal Restlessness Scale: Performance of college students with and without ADHD." *Journal of Learning Disabilities,* July–August 2003: 382–89.

Whalen, Carol K., et al. "The ADHD spectrum and everyday life: Experience sampling of adolescent moods, activities, smoking, and drinking." *Child Development,* January–February 2002: 209–27.

Wilens, Timothy E. "AOD use and attention-deficit/hyperactivity disorder." *Alcohol Health & Research World,* Spring 1998: 127–30.

Wilens, Timothy, et al. "ADHD treatment with once-daily OROS methylphenidate: interim 12–month results from a long-team open-label study." *Journal of the American Academy of Child and Adolescent Psychiatry,* April 2003: 424–35.

Wilens, Timothy E., et al. "Psychiatric comorbidity and functioning in clinically referred preschool children and school-age youths with ADHD." *Journal of the American Academy of Child and Adolescent Psychiatry,* March 2002: 262–68.

Willoughby, Michael T. "Developmental course of ADHD symptomatology during the transition from childhood to adolescence: a review with recommendations." *Journal of Child Psychology and Psychiatry and Allied Disciplines,* January 2003: 88–106.

Willy, Mary E., et al. "A study of compliance with FDA (Food and Drug Administration) recommendations for pemoline. (Cylert[R])." *Journal of the American Academy of Child and Adolescent Psychiatry,* July 2002: 785–90.

Wolke, Dieter; Patrizia Rizzo; and Sarah Woods. "Persistent infant crying and hyperactivity problems in middle childhood." *Pediatrics,* June 2002: 1054–60.

Wolraich, Mark L., et al. "Teachers' screening for attention-deficit/hyperactivity disorder: comparing multinational samples on teacher ratings of ADHD." *Journal of Abnormal Child Psychology,* August 2003: 445–55.

Wolraich, Mark L. "The use of psychotropic medications in children: an American view." *Journal of Child Psychology and Psychiatry and Allied Disciplines,* February 2003: 159–68.

Young, Karen. "Lexicor offers additional tool to help in ADHD diagnosis." *Diagnostics & Imaging Week,* March 25, 2004: 2–3.

WEBSITES

ADDvance: A Resource for Women and Girls with Attention-Deficit Disorders

Internet: www.addvance.com

An organization whose purpose is to raise awareness about AD/HD in girls and women.

A.D.D. Warehouse

300 Northwest 70th Avenue, Suite 102
Plantation, FL 33317
Phone: (800) 233-9273 or (954) 792-8100
Fax: (954) 792-8545

Internet: www.addwarehouse.com

A large distributor of books, games, videos, and other materials on AD/HD for parents and professionals.

AdhdNews.com
P.O. Box 1596
Pleasanton, CA 94566
Internet: www.adhdnews.com
A website that offers advice to parents of AD/HD children.

American Academy of Child and Adolescent Psychiatry
3615 Wisconsin Avenue, NW
Washington, DC 20016-3007
Phone: (202) 966-7300
Fax: (202) 966-2891
Internet: www.aacap.org
A professional organization for child and adolescent psychiatrists.

American Academy of Neurology
1080 Montreal Avenue
Saint Paul, MN 55116
Phone: (800) 879-1960 or (651) 695-2717
Fax: (651) 695-2791
Internet: www.aan.com
A professional organization for neurologists.

American Academy of Pediatrics
141 Northwest Point Boulevard
Elk Grove Village, IL 60007-1098
Phone: (847) 434-4000
Fax: (847) 434-8000
Internet: www.aap.org
A professional organization for pediatricians.

American Coaching Association
P.O. Box 353
Lafayette Hill, PA 19144
Phone: (610) 825-8572
Internet: www.americoach.org
An organization that provides parents with coaching specialists.

American Medical Association
515 N. State Street
Chicago, IL 60610
Phone: (800) 621-8335
Internet: www.ama-assn.org
A professional organization for physicans.

American Psychiatric Association
1000 Wilson Boulevard, Suite 1825
Arlington, VA 22209-3901
Phone: (703) 907-7300
Internet: www.psych.org
A professional organization for psychiatrists.

Attention-Deficit Information Network
58 Prince Street
Needham, MA 02492
Phone: (781) 455-9895
Internet: www.addinfonetwork.com
An organization founded by parents to offer support to other AD/HD families.

Attention Research Update
Internet: www.helpforadd.com
A free e-mail newsletter that regularly provides information on AD/HD to parents and professionals.

Belle Curve Records Inc.
Sensory Resources
2500 Chandler Avenue, Suite 3
Las Vegas, NV 89120-4064

Phone: (702) 433-0404 or (888) 357-5867
Fax: (702) 891-8899
Internet: www.bellecurve.com
Sells books and audiotapes about sensory issues.

Children and Adults with Attention-Deficit/Hyperactivity Disorder (CHADD)
8181 Professional Place, Suite 15D
Landover, MD 20785
Phone: (301) 306-7070 or (800) 233-4050
Fax: (301) 306-7090
Internet: www.chadd.org
A professional organization dedicated to improving the lives of people with AD/HD.

The Council for Exceptional Children
1110 North Glebe Road, Suite 300
Arlington, VA 22201-5704
Phone: (703) 620-3660 or (888) CEC-SPED
Fax: (703) 264-9494
Internet: www.cec.sped.org
A professional organization dedicated to improving education for people with disabilities or the gifted.

Developmental Delay Resources
4401 East West Highway, Suite 207
Bethesda, MD 20814
Phone: (301) 652-2263
Fax: (301) 652-9133
Internet: www.devdelay.org
A nonprofit organization for parents, professionals, and educators who work with special-needs children.

Federation of Families for Children's Mental Health
1101 King Street, Suite 420
Alexandria, VA 22314

Phone: (703) 684-7710

Fax: (703) 836-1040

Internet: www.ffcmh.org

A nonprofit organization that helps families of children with mental health disorders.

HEATH Resource Center

The George Washington University

2121 K Street, NW, Suite 220

Washington, DC 20037

Phone: (202) 973-0904 or (800) 544-3284

Fax: (202) 973-0908

E-mail: askheath@heath.gwu.edu

Internet: www.heath.gwu.edu

A national clearinghouse for information about college education and policies for people with disabilities.

Job Accommodation Network

P.O. Box 6080

Morgantown, WV 26506-6080

Phone (United States): (800) 526-7234 or (800) ADA-WORK

Phone (worldwide): (304) 293-7186

Fax: (304) 293-5407

Internet: www.jan.wvu.edu

A free consulting organization designed to answer questions about employment issues for those with disabilities.

KidsHealth

Internet: www.kidshealth.org

Website for families about children's health.

Learning Disabilities Association of America

4156 Library Road

Pittsburgh, PA 15234-1349

Phone: (412) 341-1515

Fax: (412) 344-0224

Internet: www.ldanatl.org
A nonprofit organization for people with learning disabilities, their families, and professionals.

Mayo Clinic Attention-Deficit Quiz
Internet: www.mayohealth.org
Online AD/HD quiz to test for the disorder in children (parent completes the quiz) or adults with possible AD/HD.

NAMI (formerly National Alliance for the Mentally Ill)
Colonial Place Three
2107 Wilson Boulevard, Suite 300
Arlington, VA 22201-3042
Phone: (703) 524-7600
Fax: (703) 524-9094
Member Services: (800) 950-NAMI
Internet: www.nami.org
A nonprofit organization for families of people with mental disorders.

National Association of Private Schools for Exceptional Children
1522 K Street, NW, Suite 1032
Washington, DC 20005
Phone: (202) 408-3338
Fax: (202) 408-3340
Internet: www.napsec.org
A nonprofit organization that helps ensure appropriate special education services for disabled individuals in both private and public sectors.

National Attention-Deficit Disorder Association
P.O. Box 543
Pottstown, PA 19464
Phone: (484) 945-2101
Fax: (610) 970-7520
Internet: www.add.org
An organization that provides information to AD/HD adults and professionals who provide services to them.

National Board for Certified Counselors
3 Terrace Way, Suite D
Greensboro, NC 27403-3660
Phone: (336) 547-0607
Internet: www.nbcc.org
A professional organization that provides certification services for counselors.

National Center for Gender Issues and ADHD
3268 Arcadia Place, NW
Washington, DC 20015
Phone: (888) 238-8588
Fax: (207) 244-9933
Internet: www.ncgiadd.org
An organization that promotes research programs and public awareness about AD/HD in girls and women.

National Center for Learning Disabilities
381 Park Avenue South, Suite 1401
New York, NY 10016
Phone: (212) 545-7510 or (888) 575-7373
Fax: (212) 545-9665
Internet: www.ld.org
An organization dedicated to research, advocacy, public awareness, and educational programs about learning disabilities.

National Information Center for Children and Youth with Disabilities
P.O. Box 1492
Washington, DC 20013-1492
Phone: (800) 695-0285
Internet: www.kidsource.com
An information and referral center that provides free information on disabilities and disability-related issues.

National Institute of Mental Health
6001 Executive Boulevard, Room 8184
MSC 9663
Bethesda, MD 20892-9663
Phone: (301) 443-4513
Internet: www.nimh.nih.gov
A federal agency dedicated to research about mental health disorders.

National Resource Center on AD/HD
(Operated by CHADD and the Centers for Disease Control
and Prevention)
8181 Professional Place, Suite 150
Landover, MD 20785
Phone: (800) 233-4050
Internet: www.help4adhd.org
A national clearinghouse of information about AD/HD.

Parent Advocacy Coalition for Educational Rights
8161 Normandale Boulevard
Minneapolis, MN 55437
Phone: (952) 838-9000 or (800) 537-2237
Fax: (952) 838-0199
Internet: www.pacer.org
A parent advocacy group for children with disabilities.

Sensory Comfort
Internet: www.sensorycomfort.com
Sells items for those with sensory processing difficulties.

Sensory Integration International
(Sponsored by The Kid Foundation)
1901 West Littleton Boulevard
Littleton, CO 80120
Phone: (310) 320-9986
Internet: www.sinetwork.org

An organization to help identify those with learning disabilities and sensory integration dysfunction, as well to promote the development of research programs.

Surgeon General
Office of the Surgeon General
5600 Fishers Lane, Room 18-66
Rockville, MD 20857
Internet: www.surgeongeneral.gov
The surgeon general's official website about public health issues.

Technical Assistance Alliance for Parent Centers
Alliance Coordinating Office
PACER Center
8161 Normandale Boulevard
Minneapolis, MN 55437-1044
Phone: (952) 838-9000
Fax: (952) 838-0199
Internet: www.taalliance.org
A project funded by the U.S. Department of Education to provide training and information to parents of children with disabilities.

Index